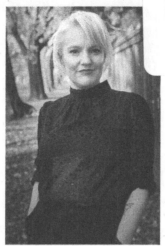

T0359422

Jacinta Parsons is a radio broadcaster and writer. She currently hosts Afternoons, a three-hour magazine show on ABC Radio Melbourne, after kicking off her radio-life at community station 3RRR and as music director across ABC Local Radio nationally with Double J. In 2020, she hosted a three-part science documentary series for ABC TV, *How to Live Younger*.

Jacinta released her first book, *Unseen: The secret world of chronic illness*, in 2020. She is an ambassador for the Crohn's and Colitis Association of Australia. She is an active member of the arts and music community and is a board member for Melbourne disability theatre company Rollercoaster.

Praise for *A Question of Age*

'It's hard to explain the relief one feels when an author tells the truth like this. This is a work of love.'
Clare Bowditch

'Deep, honest, beautiful'
Julia Zemiro

'Heartfelt, deeply thoughtful, blazing with truth-filled rage'
Peggy Frew

'At once lyrical and searing, *A Question of Age* is a book of both power and vulnerability. A uniquely honest take on what it is to age in a woman's body; how age deconstructs us, and how we can also see it as a rebuilding, and a reinvention, it is the perfect antidote to the relentless stream of sexism and ageism that women ultimately contend with. Furious, lyrical, tender and ultimately inspiring, Jacinta takes us on a journey of liberation; a tour of what it is to be a woman, and to cross over into midlife and beyond. This is a book that should be read by all women, whatever their age.'
Monica Dux

'A life-affirming and necessary read, Jacinta Parson's illumination of womankind devours our female silence and complicity, replacing it with a mediation on our impermanence that makes space for a fierce quietening, in order to hear the inner voice guiding us home. I was equal parts proud and appalled, validated and illuminated – this book gets personal and goes deep into our collective female experience, I could not look away. Confronting, nurturing, heartbreaking and uplifting, all at once – a beautifully woven insight providing a blueprint for embracing the inevitable.'
Mimi Kwa

A
Question
of Age

Jacinta
Parsons
A
Question
of Age

Women, ageing
and the forever self

ABC
BOOKS

The ABC 'Wave' device is a trademark of the
Australian Broadcasting Corporation and is used
under licence by HarperCollins*Publishers* Australia.

HarperCollins*Publishers*
Australia • Brazil • Canada • France • Germany • Holland • India
Italy • Japan • Mexico • New Zealand • Poland • Spain • Sweden
Switzerland • United Kingdom • United States of America

HarperCollins acknowledges the Traditional Custodians
of the land upon which we live and work, and pays respect
to Elders past and present.

First published in Australia in 2022
by HarperCollins*Publishers* Australia Pty Limited
Gadigal Country
ABN 36 009 913 517
harpercollins.com.au

A catalogue record for this book is available from the National Library of Australia

ISBN 978 0 7333 4216 5 (paperback)
ISBN 978 1 4607 1449 2 (ebook)

Cover design by Sandy Cull, gogoGingko
Cover images: woman's figure by Sergey Filimonov/stocksy.com/3834025; painting
on woman's body and spine of book by Peter Barritt / Alamy Stock Photo; painting on
woman's head by incamerastock / Alamy Stock Photo
Author photo by Matthew Parsons
Typeset in Bembo Std by Kirby Jones
Printed and bound in Australia by McPherson's Printing Group

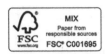

For Mika,
And your wild heart and ferocious mind.

You and I are not new,
Rather, the continuation of some other, long-ago-told love story.

I pay my respects to the Traditional Custodians of the lands and waters of the Wurundjeri Woi Wurrung people of the Kulin Nation where I live, write and work. I pay my respects also to the Traditional Custodians of the lands and waters of the Gunditjmara people, where I wrote some of this book.

I acknowledge that the colonisation of this country has attempted to destroy First Nations culture with systems that advantage white culture and directly disadvantage and harm First Nations women and their families. I acknowledge ageing for Aboriginal and Torres Strait Islander women is burdened by an inequity in healthcare, generational trauma and an over-representation of our First Nations women and their families in the criminal justice system due to inherent systemic racism. I acknowledge the strength, resilience and the relationship First Nations women have always had, and will always have, with this land.

CONTENTS

Prologue Chaos: Before We Began   1

Part 1   Fire: Casting the Woman   7
Fire: Introduction   9
Chapter 1   Cast in Fire: The Maiden   13
Chapter 2   Radiant Heat: Sluts   31
Chapter 3   Rubbed in Ash: Invisibility   42
Chapter 4   Fire Inside: The Mother   52
Chapter 5   Burnt at the Stake: The Witch   71

Part 2   Air: The Wind Cries   83
Air: Introduction   85
Chapter 6   The Trade Winds: Body   90
Chapter 7   Stillness: Midlife   103
Chapter 8   Sirocco: Mirror, Mirror   117
Chapter 9   Beaufort: The Scale   133

Part 3   Water: Parched   145
Water: Introduction   147
Chapter 10 Under Water: Secrets   154
Chapter 11 Currents: Blood   173
Chapter 12 Tsunami: Work   186
Chapter 13 Abyssal Plain: Friendship, Love, Regret   198

Part 4   Earth: Endings   205

Earth: Introduction   207

Chapter 14 Buried: Mind   213

Chapter 15 Kairos: Time   226

Chapter 16 Autolysis: Returning   234

Chapter 17 Boötes Void: Liminality   251

Epilogue   Aether: New Beginnings   261

Endnotes   269

References   281

Acknowledgements   283

This book is full of my questions of age. Questions that are influenced and limited by my perspective as a white cisgendered woman who has been advantaged by a system that has actively disadvantaged people who are queer, First Nations and/or women of colour – people who have a much greater likelihood of encountering high levels of discrimination as they age. While my identity as a disabled woman has given me an insight into some aspects of disability, and this book makes a serious endeavour to see beyond my own lived experience, I am committed to actively listening, learning, reflecting and challenging to fight for a feminism that is truly intersectional.

Chaos: Before We Began

THIS IS NOT A self-help book. Or a helpful book, necessarily.

No one really needs 'help' with ageing. It will happen no matter what we do – we have been ageing since we first cried out in this world. When I was young, I would look at ageing as some kind of oddity as I traced my finger along the lines on the faces of my grandparents. 'Who are these strange people?' I wondered.

I noticed that I was transforming into something new. That I had slowed down and that my face had changed. What was strange to me was that I didn't feel much different on the inside. Nothing felt like I thought it might. There is no sense that suddenly you change at a fundamental level and become someone who is older – someone else.

I noticed a while ago that I was becoming see-through, like I have always imagined ghosts to be. And so I took it upon myself to find ways to lessen the impact of what happens when you are an ageing woman. I bought new creams and highlighting dust so that my skin wouldn't look as tired. And I was quietly terrified of what I believed I would be forced to become.

We have been taught to be repulsed, frightened and ashamed by the prospect of ageing. Older people, middle-aged people, people older than 'youth' experience ageing in a western society as a barrier and a deficit. We have internalised ageism, and we confront it in the world around us every single day of our lives. Ashton Applewhite, one of the leading activists speaking out about ageism, believes that we have been active in the discrimination against our future selves: 'With ageism, we have internalised it. We have been complicit in our own marginalisation and it will require active consciousness-raising to correct that.'[1]

I am no better, of course. I have othered older women and quietly prayed that my skin would defy the inevitability of sagging. I was wary of the women who surely must have always been like this: Old. Tired. Sick. Angry. How could *my* self ever become like that? It was inconceivable to consider such a fundamental shift from the me as a young person and the me that would one day be old. How does it happen, this shift?

But now that I'm embarking on it, I want to sink down into ageing, to find a way to reconcile with the past that has brought me to the start of this process. To understand how I was made so I can unmake myself in time to live the life that perhaps I should be living.

This is not a book that will ask you to reclaim your life, now that you have been discarded on the scrap heap. Nor will it tell you to scream into the void where you now reside, that ageing doesn't matter. You're right, of course, it doesn't matter, but not for the reasons they force us to claim. Rather, it doesn't matter because the way we've been taught to think about ageing is a lie.

This is not a book to guide you through these stages of ageing. We will all do this in our own way and in our own time. We may skip stages, do some twice or thrice, or stay in one stage until we die.

This book will not ask you to love your lines. Or to post on social media that you feel privileged to age. Of course, this is all true; it truly *is* a privilege to age. This book primarily endeavours to understand our rage. Why, as women get older, do some of us seem to get really fucking mad? It doesn't seem to take much, if you push us even slightly, to find ourselves wanting to flip the fucking table (metaphorically, of course). I was beginning to understand that the rage I felt as I aged could not be separated from how it felt to live as a younger version of this person.

This is not simply a rage fuelled by the hormonal changes that I am yet again undertaking, this time through perimenopause and the state of menopause. I had long been told that I was wild and that when the force of fertility left my body I would become wilder. But surely this is a lie. This is not the source of my rage. It is something else altogether.

I want to trace a line back through my life to see if I can find where this all began.

* * *

When telling people that I was writing a book on ageing, I have mostly been in receipt of an incredulous 'but what would *you* know?' eyebrow or two. It is true — what *would* I know about ageing? This book is not about knowing; I am only at the early stages of what ageing will mean to me. Rather, this book is about asking how I might endeavour to do this well. Properly well. Not the kind of well that you might do if you want to overcome it or rise above it.

This is a meditation that is informed by my own experience as a white cisgendered woman from the often-obscured vantage point of the middle. The point in life when you perhaps have not yet hardened your bones to what might lay ahead. You see a blank canvas when imagining what this ageing self might look like. You have not yet been bestowed with the full golden cup of wisdom that has been promised as you cross this older person threshold, but you have begun the journey of loss, change and deep meditation on this.

For me, the landscape around ageing is not yet clear. How do I do it well and not get sucked further into the seemingly inevitable relationship with myself as a social and cultural utility?

For much of our lives, the relentless objectification we have experienced has coerced us into believing that we knew what a woman should look like since we were old enough to saunter down that road in just the right way. So just how does this pressure to conform impact the way we might see ourselves as older women? Who do we feel we need to become now?

To have lived as a woman we have functioned for the purpose of sexual gratification or for nurturing — or both, simultaneously. The maiden, the mother, the crone: the three supposed stages of our lives neatly packaged into archetypes that render us useful … or not.

After writing this book, though, I don't think I even know what it really is to be described as old. We are always getting 'older', but when do we get 'old'? And who and what determines that you are now such a beast? It is clear that it is damaging to see the world through the binary of old and young.

There has been a slew of literature written about the positive aspects of ageing, and that has an important place, but it demands that we arrive at acceptance immediately. I am interested instead in the time needed to reflect on ageing and to push back against the lies that we've been told. To grieve, to be mad, to work out what the hell has happened. I am interested to understand how, for many women, getting old is dangerous.

This book is a clarion call to rise up and burn the building. To refuse to continue to maintain it. This book wants to demand that our girls do not inherit the silence and shame of living in this way.

In this book, I am created by the elemental forces that live within me and outside of me. The forces that mess with the neutrality of life to make sure that we are subjected to change and renewal. From droughts to floods to fires, from birth to death, these are the conditions in which the human is forged.

In the fire, water, air and earth, I want to ask the question of age.

ELEMENT:

Fire

Casting the Woman

Fire

Introduction

I FIRST HAD A sense of the colour and heat of fire when I was eight years old. It was the day that would become known as Ash Wednesday. It was a day when the humidity in Melbourne made it hard to breathe. Sweat poured from my skin as I sat in our weatherboard house in front of the oscillating fan that hummed in a panic, trying in vain to neutralise a 43°C day.

On that Wednesday, 16 February 1983, there was a warning in the stillness. The feeling of danger hummed under the sounds of our regular day as fires grew around the states of Victoria and South Australia. We were hundreds of kilometres away in the city, and I was too young to understand, but I felt the danger unsettle me as I watched my parents listening to the news on the radio.

The wind came from the north, screaming down the Hume like a road train, hot and fast, gusts reaching over a hundred kilometres per hour. Suddenly, on nightfall, it changed direction and south-westerly winds sent a firestorm through Victorian and South Australian towns and lives. The city of Melbourne was surrounded, trapped by a fire that looked to ring the perimeter.

Forty-seven people in Victoria died. Twenty-eight in South Australia.

We saw photos of what was left. Most of the time it was just a chimney surrounded by rubble, as if fire somehow knows how to look after its own.

There have been other fires in my life. Those fires form part of this story.

* * *

There must have been a moment, or even a particular year, when I stopped being young and they suddenly thought of me as old. Or at least 'older'. But try as I may, it's hard to put my finger on exactly when it happened. It's difficult to know, because 'not being young' isn't quantified by an easy metric such as reaching a certain age. It's an ephemera. Or perhaps a witchcraft.

One of the first stages of getting older was the experience of becoming invisible. Or perhaps see-through, like a body of water you dive into with only your eyes trying to see to the bottom. When it first happened, I didn't understand how I was suddenly rendered not of this world. And then, when I understood I had been discarded, I didn't know how to respond to this kind of disappearance.

The moment when I became invisible happened surprisingly suddenly as a deliberate act of erasure. As the mafia would say, I had been 'disappeared'. Out of sight, out of mind.

To understand how I disappeared, I knew I must go back to the beginning, to the day when I was first cast in the fire. A day, millions of years ago, when I was formed. The iron cast cut around my heart and mind, when my dreams were made from me. It's the same cast that people like me have been fired in for eternity. We have been built as this idea of woman. I had been made from the same mould in the same way that many women have been made. I had the same story of those who have been loved and mourned, who were tortured and hunted and burnt.

I am not new. Instead, I am the continuation of a certain kind of story. A story that has been on an eternal loop. I have been subjected to the same fate as so many women before me – to be lost on this earth. And then to be found again, but different.

I was cast in the same fire that was first lit by my ancestors. And now I want to understand the story that I am continuing. I understand more keenly now that I harbour a life force, a secret key to the worlds that have existed before me. I know about my ancestors in the way my breath moves, in and out, in and out. I am riddled with the pain and the imaginations of the lives that live within me. Lives that I might only know by the way my head tilts slightly, just as my great-great-great-grandmother may have tilted hers.

* * *

Fire is where this story begins, the place where I start to look for answers about how I might age. In the ash and the heat. In the embers and the smoke. In what it might mean to be reborn again from the razing as new life shoots from the stillness, from the blackness.

11

I want to understand how age is going to impact me and what it means for me to live inside a body that changes, that is changed and that makes it difficult to live as simply as I might want. When did this change happen? And is it possible, as a woman, to speak about it as a shared experience with other women?

I am spending more and more time thinking about what ageing will mean. How I will be transformed. How well I might adapt. How much change I can withstand before I try to alter it somehow, to push back. How vulnerable I will become. But also, will I now be free?

I know that I must go back to the beginning, to the time when they tricked me into believing that I was indeed new, to find out just how they convinced me to disappear.

The fire is where I am cast and it is the rage that burns inside my belly.

Fire

CHAPTER 1

Cast in Fire:
The Maiden

I WATCHED HIM PLACE the glass in the furnace. 'As hot as Hades,' he said as it heated up to two thousand degrees. Impossible to imagine that anything can survive that type of heat. The heat changes the shape of the glass and transforms it into something that can be worked with so it can become something new, something that he was already imagining. 'People have been blowing glass since around the first century BC,' he tells me, his eyes on the gob of glass that he is pulling out of the furnace. Soon enough, this simple lump would be blown and transformed into something almost unrecognisable. Something beautiful.

* * *

I walked to the strip of shops down the hill and along the main road. Lined up like a gang of scruffy children were a milk bar, a fishmonger and a computer parts store. They were covered in a grime that had been layering for years, and the once proud white paint had soiled to grey. I had three dollars tucked into my jeans to spend on some salt and vinegar chips and maybe a chocolate Big M.

I took this walk as much as I could. I was fourteen, bored and desperate to feel my skin against the world. I hungered to find myself somewhere new, or at least I wanted to be new myself.

I was dressed for the occasion, my favourite singlet top with the tiny flowers and the new white jeans that my mum had bought me. I had teased my fringe up and flipped it over so that there was a quiff at the front so that it looked like I had more hair than I did. I did the best I could with the tiny amount of makeup I had hidden in the bottom of my bathroom drawers, just enough so that no one would notice.

And sitting on top of my skin I would wear a vulnerability that burnt when the wind blew across it. 'Shhhh,' I would hiss. 'Hold it together, you idiot.'

My entry into this world happened, it seemed, when I had not been watching. I had sensed it coming, I think, when it was just rolling in over the hill. But I didn't understand what it would be like to be part of this new world. My teenage performance so far had been a hopeful shot in the dark for something I wasn't sure about. What would it mean to be loved?

I spent hours daydreaming in a dark bedroom. I would close the door, like a caterpillar taking to its cocoon. Closing my eyes to the transformation that was taking place within me. I would imagine what might emerge when the transition was complete. I squeezed my eyes shut, hoping that when they sprang open I would be different. Beautiful. Wild.

I studied other girls in my year at school like a naturalist observes the behaviour of plants. What had those girls conjured to look as they did? Their hair so perfectly placed. Their eyes dewy and alive. Their clothing a perfect measure of rebellion and attraction. How was it that they performed this transition into the world with such confidence? Who told them how to make this change seem so effortless? Their leaves twisting and turning, knowing instinctively that they needed to follow the light. How were they taught to intuit the path of the sun?

The older women weren't much help. I heard their whispers and giggles, surely enacting a shared ritual of horror masked in play at what might be ahead for us as we entered their world. I felt their eyes upon us as they observed that our bodies were beginning to look more like theirs. There was fear in those eyes, because now that we looked like them, there were secrets they knew they should share. There were whispered stories here and there about things that didn't really matter, but they didn't share the most violent secrets, the ones that we should have been told. Those secrets remained held within lips that had calcified with silence, becoming still like stone.

I felt the gap between the old women (anyone over thirty years old) and us young girls widen as they tried and failed to bring us safely into their world. We should have known their secrets before we painted our lips and hoped to be loved. Why didn't they tell us? Why don't we now tell little girls what it's like to live like this? To be watched. To grow old. To carry such pain and to experience such enormous pleasure.

I have hidden my own secrets. And kept my own silence. Many times.

The old women hid their discomfort, too, by laughing at our attempts to fit in. 'Gee, you've spent enough time doing your hair, haven't you? Who are you trying to look pretty for, hey?' But under their laughter sounded a warning, an alarm that told us we were foolish to even think of ourselves this way. Underneath their words sat the real meaning: 'You're only going to get hurt.'

Were they trying to protect us from what lay ahead in this new world? Or did our likeness trigger a hatred that brewed somewhere deep inside?

The old women would talk about us while we were within earshot, like we were toddlers unable to understand what was being said. They would point out the bodies that had developed too fast. Or the ones whose clothing revealed too much skin.

They knew those girls would be dangerous if they had ideas about what they might do with those bodies. These were the bad girls, unafraid of showing their skin to this hungry new world. I was cautioned to keep away from those ones – they were asking for it. Sluts.

And silently, almost through some sort of secret code, the old women shared the shame of inheriting what it was to be a woman. We have been passing our shame from one generation to the other, hidden like a stowaway inside our skin. The tugging embarrassment of its shape. The discomfort of the attention that it receives. Its power. Its allure. Its destruction. Its pain. Its pleasure.

* * *

Recently, the walk to the shops had changed. I could feel the rumble, a vibration under my feet, but couldn't quite tell where it was coming from. The energy had shifted around me. The change was small to begin with. Like the way air starts to feel heavy all over you when it's about to rain. Or when you notice that the ants are changing direction, frantically returning home.

But something was different. Something imperceptible had shifted. The wind had swung around and changed direction, and the fire front was now heading towards me.

The changes in my body had laid a pathway to a new world. Men had started to notice me. Men who had an uncanny ability to break your daydream and make you look back at them. The older men, with fat stomachs and broken teeth, would make a small noise so you'd look up. And then they'd smile and look you straight in the eye. 'You're beautiful, baby.'

They were masterful at the game they had likely been playing for decades. Their words would twist and travel down my spine like a current, warning me that there was danger somewhere close. The same words that might have been innocent coming out of another mouth, but here, dripping off their fat lips, you could smell violence on their breath, coiled up tight and ready to explode.

At first I would jump in fright. I had been lost in other thoughts, the kinds of thoughts a child might have before she knows that it's not safe to daydream anymore. I might have been lost in how the trees moved in the wind. How the smell of eucalyptus swings on a current of air.

Soon enough, the calling on the street became so familiar that I had started to expect it. Like an animal watching, I had become alert to it, trying to sense even the tiniest change in my environment that would suggest it was about to happen. And slowly and quietly, I had become hopeful for it. Reliant on it.

Sometimes I would catch his eye before he had caught mine. If he didn't look, or call at me from his car, I wondered what I had done wrong. If the boys on the bus didn't make comments as I got on, did they think I was ugly? Were my legs too fat?

I watched as other girls were yelled at. Whistled. Tooted. And wondered what they had that day that I didn't. I would try to see them as the men saw them. I shifted my gaze and wondered what it would be like to feel desire for these bodies. And I learnt to look at the world like these men might. I learnt to see *myself* as these men might.

I noticed that it wasn't just young women or teenagers who were being catcalled. I was fourteen when I was first whistled at like a dog, but for many girls catcalling starts much younger. Girls as young as eleven are being pulled out of their daydreams and forced to enter a new world.[1]

I watched as young girls looked around them, confused, trying to make sense of what was happening. What did it mean to be treated like this? How do you explain the feeling of shame that is now alive in you? Suddenly being forced to see yourself through the prism of desire and power, you find yourself lost in a foreign land, scrambling to learn the language. And this idea of you, born in the mind of someone on the street, suddenly has the power to disrupt your childish play. It doesn't feel right anymore to continue pretending with doll's houses. The climbing of trees. Colouring for hours with pencils.

Nine out of ten women have experienced catcalling or street harassment. And of those nine women, half were still children the first time it happened. Absurdly, the catcalling of our girls is normalised as part of the experience of growing up. When I was growing up, it was expected to happen. It was inevitable.

Street harassment is fundamentally about entitlement. A birthright. It isn't necessarily about acquiring power but rather asserting that the right to our bodies has already been won. When you realise, as a young girl, that you have already been acquired, it's a game that you realise you quickly need to learn how to play. You know that the world you are inhabiting is not yours except to learn the rules so you might avoid harm.

What is played out on the streets is about many things, including testing boundaries. When street harassment is normalised it becomes a necessary rite of passage for some men to enact as a public show. Men are performing their entitlement to possess women for the benefit of each other. Men show each other that they are unafraid to claim what is rightfully theirs. Often this is done together, in packs. We perform our way to misogyny. And when that performance is normalised and left unchallenged, we all believe that it is somehow inevitable. That we are powerless against it.[2]

Coming across those packs of men, my heart would quicken. I had been told: 'Don't look down. Look ahead, like you're not scared.' There seemed to be nothing that might allow escape from some sort of exchange. Like wolves that prowl together, using their eyes and ears for each other, a pack of men is often operating under one system. There is a hierarchy that is automatically enforced, and each member or the pack naturally takes their place.[3]

I knew they were laughing at things that were not meant for us to hear. This kind of power is found in the unspoken rules of their game. They know we can't hear what they say about our breasts or what they'd like to do to us, or that we're dogs, or sluts – and that's part of the thrill. That we are walking in front of them, oblivious to the abuse, is part of the game. It is the performance of power.

I have heard some men say that they worry about their daughters or the women they are close to because they 'know what men are like'. How is it, I have often wondered, that you know this about men? Have you been part of those packs, those groups of men who wanted to rip right through a girl? But I know all the men you know, so who is it that you've heard speaking like this? When is it that you have been inside one of these huddles to hear the things that are said about women? And what did you do?

Danny Blay has been working to understand violence against women for decades. Working in different roles to educate men about how violence is perpetuated in our communities, he has facilitated a number of programs where men are offered the opportunity to see the impact of their behaviour on the world around them and given the tools for change.

'Men are often caught in the same trap as women. The same way women feel that they must go along with the demeaning sexualised behaviour focused on them, men feel that they can't rock the boat. The group performance can sometimes be about the power of gendered expectations. If a man or boy speaks out against the group, there are serious consequences. It's much easier to go along with what the group wants to do,' he tells me.

'Boys and men have learnt that they can objectify women, and sometimes they feel they should objectify women, because that's what real boys and real men do.

Boys not participating with the other boys when they're

hooning around their bikes and catcalling girls – if they're not participating in that, what's that going to mean to them socially? What's it going to mean for them for their own identity? Their own sense of self? So the act of catcalling girls and women isn't in isolation. It's an exertion of power. And it's a demonstration to the other boys and men that "I'm a bloke and I'm a real boy. And don't question me ..."'

He has found that there is a resistance to seeing themselves in this way. 'The vast majority of boys and men do not want to even consider that they play a role in the subject of occasional objectification of women.'

The change, Blay believes, needs to come from men themselves, calling it out. Facing up to the collective male agenda and owning solutions.[4]

Catcalling was the practical and public assertion that women belonged to men, and street harassment existed so we didn't forget. Catcalls ensured we never relaxed, were never complacent, that we never felt entirely safe. The whistles and comments were targeted so that they would land straight under our skin, so that no matter how brave you might feel, you always understood just how vulnerable you were.

It was the mid-eighties and we were on the brink of a third wave of feminism. A white feminism asserting that (certain) women could 'have it all' was slowly and finally making its way to the lower socio-economic swamps of Australia. In the suburb where I lived, where white lower middle-class mediocrity was nurtured, white feminism had taught us that it was insulting to be objectified like this, to be the interest of a male's lazy gaze. To be subjected to his animal desires and to accept them, or, worse, to comply.

I understood early on that I should object to being treated without care for the mind and the heart that beat ferociously inside me. I was told I should work hard to dismantle the patriarchal project. That young white women especially, who could find an adjacent benefit to the white male power, should resist the cunning ways that it might recruit. Do not giggle. Do not smile. Do not dress to please. Resist the lure of its power.

But it wasn't possible to heed these instructions then. I quickly understood that to survive, I needed to learn how to play this game.

There has always been a violence in the demand for woman to be monocultural and mono-structural, to be a single version of a physiology and a psychology. Women have always been controlled this way, developing limited notions in the expression of what it feels and looks like to be considered a woman while we are dominated by our need to placate and console the male gaze.

We adopted ideas of the woman and did the work on our own oppression by inflicting these ideas upon ourselves and each other. We were told we should want larger breasts, smaller waists and pure skin. I didn't ever feel like a woman, not really. Not the idea of woman that had been depicted on every billboard or TV show since I was a child. I always felt like there were lessons on femininity that I had been absent for. Where did women learn how to wear makeup and high heels and clothing that enhanced their bodies? How did they feel so comfortable with the ways of being women together – the secrets, the closeness?

On Australian streets, the bodies most likely considered 'women' are concepts born post-colonisation from a white cultural idea of womanhood. Women who are white and perform a brand of femininity that is petite and compliant fit this construction. While all women endured oppression via patriarchal systems, women of colour and First Nations women also had to endure the violence of colonisation and imperialism. White women have been agents and complicit in the colonisation and othering of First Nations women. The 'other' women outside the colonial model would be either fetishised or nullified.

It is something that Aakanksha Manjunath, founder and executive director of It's Not A Compliment, knows something about. Through its research and campaigns on the realities of street harassment, the organisation has found that vulnerable people – often anyone who could be coded as 'other' – were more likely to experience additional layers of harassment. 'I think women of colour don't actually enjoy public spaces in the same way that white women do,' says Manjunath. 'And also this idea of what it is like to be considered "true Australians"; a woman of colour is less likely to enjoy the freedoms of being a full Australian compared to a white woman.'[5]

Natasha Sharma works on the data side of things as a research and policy officer at It's Not A Compliment. She describes her personal experience as having much the same trajectory as is reflected in the stats. 'I definitely experienced the peak of catcalling and street harassment around the age of fifteen or sixteen, when I would go out with my friends. It would come from forty-year-old men asking us to come join them, you know, have a drink, or come over and sit with them. Just generally, somebody will make a comment, some sort of sexual comment about your body. Even recently, I was just riding my bike to work and somebody was like, "Nice tits."'[6]

And women who didn't easily code as women – trans women, or women who didn't play to the narrow concepts of a feminine ideal – were erased, harassed or violently threatened into compliance.

A survey done by the University of New South Wales found that violence against transgender people, who are often hyper-visible, was reported by fifty per cent of the respondents as compared to only fourteen per cent of the general population.[7] This makes visibility for transgender women extremely dangerous and if you are also from a CALD background, you are nearly twenty per cent more likely to suffer multiple instances of sexual harassment than other women. The more intersecting identities, the more dangerous it is for a woman to be on the street.[8]

Young women have come to expect that the harassment will be normalised when they enter public space. Reflecting on her first experiences at bars and clubs at eighteen, Natasha says, 'You just assumed that it's very normal to be groped. And then you realise that it shouldn't actually be happening on a regular basis, but for about two years, that's just what I thought clubbing was.'[9]

* * *

There is a line that we intuit we cannot cross. Like a fire that will inexplicably travel to a point and then stop, it will burn your neighbour's house to the ground but somehow spare your own. You learn never to cross that line. Showing any disdain for the attention, for example, would render you a different sort of target. I walked around with a fear of being laughed at because I was a pig, or a dog, or a slut. A bigger group might call out and then challenge you to defy the ritual. 'What's your problem?' they would sneer. 'Can't you take a joke? Don't you like us? Bitch.'

I was average-looking at best and understood that I didn't have much currency. Oily blonde hair that was so thin it almost disappeared. Patchy skin and a large nose. I was very aware of my price and that I should be happy with whatever attention I got. I didn't have a right to argue or to act uppity or bitchy about it. Instead, I had to smile sweetly and shrug. Don't threaten. Don't argue back.

'Whatever,' we would say to each other, and roll our eyes. 'How desperate.' But secretly many of us believed it was worse if they didn't call out or whistle to us like dogs. I didn't like the walk if it was totally silent. The silence felt like its own kind of slight – like I was being forced to not exist at all.

And what we carried, like our mothers, and their mothers before them, was the belief that we were entirely responsible for our lot. Those catcalls, or the men who touched us on the train, or the ones who pushed us to the ground and hurt us, happened because we had done something to encourage it. Without our bodies taunting them there would have been no problems. What did we expect?

While my group of friends affirmed to each other that our worth was more than the experience of the men who drove past us on the street, we knew that we would never really have any power against its insidious reach. Those long tentacles would find us eventually. A girl had better learn her place or she'd be shown it soon enough.

If it didn't catch up to us then, I knew that someday it would. Those men who would call out to us from cars or look at us while they were playing with their kids in the park would also be the men who would employ us, teach us, date us, run our country, be our police, coach us, run our hospitals.

Somewhere along the line we would be forced to submit to those catcalls in the numerous forms that they manifested. Our worth was always going to be awarded to us. And when something is awarded, it can be taken away. We didn't have much say in how we might win at this.

Eyes up – watch your step, girly.

* * *

Forty-three, twenty-five, thirty-seven – the numbers that marked a woman over fifty years ago. An article in *New York Magazine* from 1968, 'Boom and bust on Wall Street' by Leonard Sloane, tells the story of Francine Gottfried. In the opening paragraph we are told of Francine's chest, waist and hip measurements and that she wears tight sweaters. We know that she arrives at the same subway station each day at 1.28 p.m. and, due to the size of her bust, has started to receive a startling amount of attention.

'Broker told broker, banker told banker, clerk told clerk to "be out there" by 1:15 each afternoon … By the third week in September, the groups had become a crowd and the crowd had become boisterous. There were applause and cheers when Francine made her 1:28 p.m. appearance … No one knew her name, but they all recognized her figure when it appeared.

'"I didn't do anything," she said over and over… "What are they doing this for?"'

The story continues that Francine's appearance from her regular train trip into Manhattan each day to start work drew such enormous attention that two New York morning papers reported her name, picture and job location, 'so it's not surprising that Friday's multitude of Francine-watchers reached a record of over 10,000'.

'"When I was 16, I looked like a woman already," Francine says. "The teachers in Eastern District High School, which I attended, started to look at me and so did the construction workers in the area. After I saw this happening, I'd just ignore it because otherwise I would smile and it could lead them on."'[10]

'Girl watching', as it was called, was a criminal offence in some parts of the United States in the twenties and thirties. In places like LA, it was made a criminal offence for 'two or more men, or boys 14 years of age or over, to ogle women in public.'[11]

A decade later and around fifteen years before Francine Gottfried was publicly humiliated, an advertising executive in New York sought to flip the perception of ogling women from being the occupation of the lower class to that of a 'mainstream, middleclass activity'. He launched a guide called *The Girl Watcher* that mirrored the way people might watch birds. To assist him in launching the book he also founded the American Society of Girl Watchers, which granted members lapel pins and guidebooks.

The guidebook is full of emphasis on body parts like legs and breasts and outlines the various ways men might find themselves in a position to watch a girl. In a 1966 edition, a caption under a photo with the leg of a woman protruding from a car door reads: 'Joe Beagin, founder of the International Society of Girl Watchers, uses the ploy of stretching his shoulder in order to leer unnoticed at a seated woman.'

One of the earlier editions breaks down vast array of girl watchers by type: 'The Flusher, The Peeker, The Stalker, The Percher, The Swivel-Head.' And the types of interests different girl watchers might have: 'The Legman, The Hipster, The Derriere Devotee, The Booze Mouse, The Lipsophile, The Nymphlover.'[12]

Francine Gottfried understood from an early age that resistance was futile and possibly dangerous. It's just a bit of fun, they mock. What's your fucking problem − are you stuck up or something? Don't you like men telling you you're beautiful?' And just like that, if anything went wrong, women were responsible. If someone got hurt, it was because the bitches didn't know their place or how to take a joke.

I was immediately fascinated by how this system worked. It wasn't women who looked a certain way, or who acted or reacted in a certain way. It was all women. Well, not all women − it was young women.

I watched from around corners. I took silent notes as I tried to understand how I fitted into it all. Would he wait until she had walked past and then turn around to watch her from behind? Would he whistle when she was just far enough away that she couldn't react to the attention and be forced to just cop it from afar? Would the married man walking with his wife look from the corner of his eye to go undetected? Would she be called to, or whistled at, or stopped and spoken to directly? 'Nice rack, bitch.'

Walking past a group of men would have its own special rules. I could feel my face heating up as I approached them. I would draw in breath and look straight ahead. 'I'm not a bitch,' I would try to cast ahead of me before I arrived in their view. 'I can have a laugh too, no worries.' There was always a current of energy that swirled around a group of men. Brace yourself. You've done this before.

At eighteen, I caught a group of boys watching one of my friends when we were camping in Byron Bay. They didn't see me watching them. At first it was their energy that caught my attention; I could smell their hunger as they stood above us on a balcony that overlooked a common area. She was beautiful. Her skin shone, her hair was long and glorious, and she was charming and fun to be around.

I would hide my body in this world. I couldn't bear that I looked the way I did. It was very clear that I wasn't beautiful, so I prepared to save myself the embarrassment of trying. 'Less is more,' one of my friends said to me as I layered up clothing to head to the beach. 'Even if you're fat, the less you have on the better.'

I could watch the world around me without much disturbance. No one was ever watching me, so I would spend hours lost. Sometimes I wouldn't notice that I had been standing still, frozen in the middle of the footpath just watching, immersed in some sort of amateur analysis of the human condition. I was endlessly fascinated by how it all worked. Is this what it was like to be desired by men? Is this what they were really like when they thought no one was watching them?

There were at least six of them on that Byron Bay balcony, jostling and moving together like a chain ran between them, and the ringleader was holding a camera. I had seen him speaking to my friend over the course of the last couple of days and he had seemed almost shy, the kind of boy you assume is sweet with his mop of brown hair, expensive teeth and full lips, and skin that flushed perfectly around a scattering of well-placed, innocent-looking freckles.

He stood at the front of the group with the camera trained on her body. 'C'mon, baby,' he said to the laughter and encouragement of the boys who milled around him. 'Smile for the camera, baby. C'mon, show us your tits.' Part of this performance was about her oblivion. A group of boys with their eyes on her body, imagining all sorts of things they would like to do to it. This is how they liked to play this game.

They were powerful because she didn't know what they were doing to her — it was their secret that they thought of women the way they did. They knew well enough that they needed to hide these sorts of blatant games from women; they knew this needed to stay between them. But there was no question from any of them whether this felt good. It did. It felt great.

He sensed something, turned and caught me watching, then immediately dropped the camera down to his waist. These rituals were not for voyeurs like me. I held his gaze. He realised he'd been caught, but it soon dawned on him that it didn't matter. Who the fuck did I think I was? Ugly bitch. He stared back at me and smiled. This was his game.

Fire

CHAPTER 2

Radiant Heat: Sluts

I ALWAYS LOVED THE feeling of heat on my legs, pushed up as close to the old Vulcan gas heater in our lounge room as I could get. As soon as the backs of my legs became unbearably warm I would spin around and warm the fronts, then continue back and forth for hours while I watched telly. The little gas pilot light would be lit at the beginning of autumn and flicker right through until summer, when we'd turn it off to clean it. And then the loud 'clack, clack' as we would try for hours to reignite the pilot flame as the sun had begun to sink in the sky.

Through the eighties we were warned about those old heaters; we'd seen news reports of dressing gowns going up in flames. 'Don't get too close to that fire,' they'd warn. 'You've seen what happens to little girls when they get too close …'

* * *

What about the young women who refused to look down and smile coyly to show they understood their place? The girls who stared straight back? The girls who weren't going to be silenced? Who had been born with the fire of their ancestors in their bellies? The ones who couldn't be sold or care less about the value men placed on them? Or the girls who dared to monetise this type of objectification, finding employment or marrying because of it? The ones who were in some way empowered via it?

But sexual empowerment of women has been considered an illegitimate and coerced form of sexual identity. When a woman plays to their objectification, we are told that because it has been constructed by the male gaze it isn't empowered. We are too stupid to understand what has been done to us.

What happened to the girls who claimed this type of objectification as theirs to own? Who found a beauty through their body as object? These girls self-objectified in ways that the rest of the world pretended to be shocked and uncomfortable with, girls who had the outrageous fortitude to say loudly, 'It's mine, and I want to see it as beautiful – I want it to be powerful, I want it to be sexual.'

Many believe that the self-objectification that takes place by women is not a form of empowerment but rather a dangerous furtherment of the toxic gaze that dominates their highly sexualised lives. There is a genuine concern for the psychological damage that this self-objectification can have for girls who mimic and enact it in play. The concern centres around what is being perpetuated about our value if we participate and propagate these images of ourselves.

And so it follows that we were interrogated by the older generation who were charged with protecting our purity. 'What were you wearing to get that sort of attention? Your skirt is too short. Your top is too low. You can't wear that out. You're asking for trouble.'

I felt the weight of that responsibility hang inside my body. I can feel the trail of embarrassment that I had pushed down so deep that I'm still finding it decades later, hidden in the dark parts of me that still somehow believe that any violation against me was, and is, my fault.

Learning early that we could be coerced to participate in such violence has quietened me. Lost was that feeling of freedom, that utterly innocent joy of closing my eyes and feeling the music rush my body, because I knew it wasn't safe – it's always just a matter of time. You will be blamed for being stupid enough to be lost in that moment. What did you expect?

It felt dangerous to walk around inside this type of body. We quickly learnt not to upset or encourage the men we knew would try to hurt us. We had to dance the line between desire and purity. To make sure you don't make them look stupid. Smile – but not too widely. Skirts – not too short, not too long.

Young bodies afford the potential acquisition of power via their corruption. There is a supposed animal thirst for them, a belief that an impossible hunger takes over the male if he is tempted by them. A desire to take a dominion over what is rightly theirs. To be the first to make the conquest. To be the first to colonise this form.

And best still, the strategy is to accuse the little girls of the crime that has been committed against them, to turn the blame back on them. You were asking for it. What were you wearing? How did you encourage this? You shouldn't have been out alone.

And yet, the argument time and time again is that the recasting of toxic concepts of objectification by women is a furtherment of the capitalist commodification of the woman, not a disruption to it.

'WAP', a 2020 hip-hop release by Cardi B featuring Megan Thee Stallion, blew up the internet on release because of its video overtly celebrating women-led sexual gratification and lyrics unwavering in their enthusiasm about a 'wet-ass pussy'. Unsurprisingly, conservative commentators expressed outrage at the assumed impact on impressionable young girls, and parents complained about girls replicating the sexualised dance moves. The condemnation also came from commentators like Russell Brand, a comedian and high-profile contemporary 'thinker' who questioned whether 'we achieve equality by aspiring to the values established by the forces or authors of the hierarchy and system itself? That is, do women achieve equality by aspiring to and replicating the values that have been established by males?' He suggested instead, in his seventeen-minute vlog, that 'WAP' wasn't revolutionary and instead just more 'capitalist objectification'.[1]

It has long been an issue when women make capital from self-objectification, as if this somehow makes it morally problematic, a critique not always levelled at anyone else who make capital from the objectification of women. An opinion piece in *The Sydney Morning Herald* argued that 'all this conjecture and debate only distracts from what I arguably dislike most about this song and that is I believe its essence isn't to liberate but to sell'.[2]

One thing is for sure, when little girls are seen to be using their objectification as an advantage, even if the advantage is momentary and not within their control, they become a serious target to destroy.

* * *

Jessica woke up early and followed her mum out to the car. Every Saturday was like this, driving silently to the Dandenong market to do the weekly shopping. She loved being in the car with her. Feeling safe without needing to say anything, knowing that she had her own jobs that her mum gave her to do when they got to the market. While her mum seemed to be safe from the sexualisation, her older sister was already seen as an object, to be harassed and persuaded. Jessica saw the way men looked at her, talked to her and followed her.

Jessica was only eleven years old when she was 'felt up' for the first time. On this Saturday morning, another weekly trip to the market, chilly, unglamorous. She wore 'weekend clothes' – shapeless items that didn't feel like they would garner attention, practical for warmth. 'I was eleven,' she says to me with incredulity. 'Eleven.' But even now, knowing how wrong it was to have been sexually assaulted at the age of eleven, she hesitates to describe it in that way. 'I guess I didn't think it was such a big deal then, but I suppose the fact I remember it all these years later suggests it must have made a big impact on me.

I felt a man touch me. He grabbed my arse – it was quick, there for a moment and then it wasn't. I turned around and he was smiling at me and so I knew something bad had happened. But in that moment, when you're so young, I don't think your brain is able to find the language for what is happening to you.

I still remember such a feeling of shame. I felt embarrassed because it happened, and I felt like it was my fault. Like I'd done something to instigate it. To encourage it. I didn't say anything. I didn't turn around and say anything to my mum – I just let it go.'

That morning she had been a little girl, with little girl ideas of the world. After that morning she understood herself differently. 'From a very early age, I clearly saw that I was a sexual object, like I could be an object of sexual gratification to someone. And I think that just kept getting reinforced.'

When she was around twelve years old she would walk home from school with her older sister. A car slowed down and circled them as they walked, full of loud and leery men in their twenties or thirties. Her sister screamed, 'She's just a kid, twelve years old. Fuck off!'

Instead of being deterred, they continued to circle. 'Show us your tits,' they screamed at her twelve-year-old body. Jessica remembers the shame and embarrassment, 'but at that point, I was older and almost wanted the sexual attention. There was part of me that felt a weird mix of pride, because it's like, oh, I am sexually interesting to someone. I must be pretty and so I have some value because I'm getting attention.'

Those conflicting feelings knocked up against each other. Deep feelings of shame and a sense of responsibility for what she felt was definitely wrong, but also a hope for sexual interest from men. 'I also perceived myself as fat, so the idea of me being fat and being wanted by someone was really exciting. But it never made me feel good. I always felt like shit about it because it was so tumultuous. At any moment, any guy could turn around after being nice to me for a sexual reason and say, "You're gross, and I don't want you anymore." In those moments, I felt such a shame, like I was selling myself for this. And it definitely impacted how early I started being sexual with people. Because I really wanted the gratification.'[3]

* * *

In the Britney Spears video '... Baby One More Time', we see one of the first depictions of the pop star who would go on to become one of the most successful musicians of our time. Sitting at a school desk staring at the clock in a conservative uniform with pink fluffy hair ties, the bell rings and she is released. In the next scene we see her dancing in front of a group of girls her age with a redesigned uniform, white collared shirt tied up to reveal a midriff and thigh-high socks. At the time of filming she was sixteen years old.

In this video, Britney Spears embodies the line teen girls are often accused of walking: complicit and manipulative in their objectification while behaving as though they are innocent to the 'trap' they have set to entice older men into illegal sexual activity with them. They must be aware of their sexual allure and therefore it is their responsibility. Older men who are enticed have been tricked.

In a 1999 article for *Rolling Stone* entitled 'Britney Spears: Inside the mind (and bedroom) of America's teen queen', the question is asked, 'Is Spears bubble gum jailbait, jaded crossover diva or malleable Stepford teen?' Without giving her much option in terms of choice, the suggestion is that she is framed entirely by her relationship to a constructed and manipulative sexuality.

The opening paragraph describes her this way: 'Britney Spears extends a honeyed thigh across the length of the sofa ...

The BABY PHAT logo of Spears' pink T-shirt is distended by her ample chest, and her silky white shorts – with dark blue piping – cling snugly to her hips. She cocks her head and smiles receptively.' The article goes on to suggest that she has set a trap: 'Admittedly, that trap is carefully baited by a debut video that shows the seventeen-year-old singer cavorting around like the naughtiest of schoolgirls. But, as Spears points out, nothing is actually revealed. "All I did was tie up my shirt!" she says … "I'm wearing a sports bra under it. Sure, I'm wearing thigh-highs, but kids wear those – it's the style."'[4]

That Spears had to defend herself against being seen as a temptress by disclosing the type of bra that she was wearing is heartbreaking. The brewing violence in the writing – the 'watch out, girly' in its tone – reveals the very real danger for young women who claim any space that might explore and empower their own imagery.

Of all the forms that women take, teen girls are both the most powerful and the most reviled. 'How vacuous and unnecessary is their art?' we mock. We sneer at how much it plays up to the male gaze and therefore is both noticed and diminished at once. 'Where would they have learnt to move their bodies like that? To perform in such a way?' Sluts.

Just how she was one of the 'naughtiest of schoolgirls' with the brimming sexual tone of danger is unclear. After rewatching the music video numerous times in the light of a twenty-year gap between that article and today, it is horrifying to see what Britney and other teens were subjected to by this commentary and subsequent treatment. Dancing in a tied-up school shirt (possibly suggesting rebellion against an education system) and moving in unison with a group of dancers behind her, Spears is then joined by a group of schoolboys in conservative uniforms who do not leer at or touch her. They simply dance with her.

It's clear that Britney was positioned as complicit in her sexual objectification when she emerged onto our televisions. The argument that persisted was that she had intended to make money off her objectification, which is still a punishable taboo. More than that, though, she was understood as having set a trap. But to trap who or what? Was it a trap for the predacious men who prowled around young girls? In any case, it became clear that she would eventually be punished.

Britney Spears was one of the 'naughty' girls, and we know what happens to bad girls who are unafraid of their own objectification or even dare to show control of their own power.

You can read the Britney story and what happened in the twenty-odd years since the release of that first video on multiple platforms. In short, she was devoured, limb by limb, and then was blamed for her own annihilation. In the light of extensive think pieces and the *New York Times* documentary *Framing Britney Spears*, we've recently started to reconcile our hatred towards young women like Spears who we so easily burnt. 'They got too close to the fire,' we use to argue.

So easily discarded and written off as unstable was Spears that she was virtually wiped from the face of the earth, dismissed for the pop music she created and for being so masterful as to understand the extent of her power with the release of her first supposedly 'hyper-sexualised' video clip. How dare she! So within the space of years, she was destroyed. Laughed at. And her fans were treated the same. This young teen girl had the treatment of the witches before her.

An Instagram post from Britney Spears in early 2021 read:

My life has always been very speculated … watched …
and judged really my whole life!!! For my sanity I need
to dance to @iamstevent every night of my life 🐌🐌🐌
to feel wild and human and alive!!! I have been exposed
my whole life performing in front of people 😳😳😳!!!
It takes a lot of strength to TRUST the universe with
your real vulnerability cause I've always been so judged …
insulted … and embarrassed by the media … and I still
am till this day 👻👻👻!!!![5]

On reflection, I realised that I also participated in the
destruction of Britney Spears. I believed them when they told
me that she was worthless. That she was losing her mind. That
she wasn't worth saving. I participated in undermining women
like her and have scoffed at teenage girls and all the things
they hold dear. I believed that my own interests were stupid,
that the only way you could truly love music was if you knew
the drummer and the year the guitar player took a break for a
cocaine habit.

I too have blood on my hands.

Jessica, who grew up with her own levels of objectification,
agrees that it wasn't until this year that she realised that she had
also been sold the story and bought into it. 'She is a perfect
example of the system of misogyny. Up until that point I
thought that, you know, she was a crazy, slutty girl, because
she brought it on herself. She's fame-hungry, power-hungry
and so she gets what she gives. Then, in the last year and a half,
I really was wondering, "Why am I buying into this narrative
when it doesn't actually make any sense?"'

So deeply internalised is my own misogyny that I believed
that girls who edged close to the fire and had been burnt had

likely done the wrong thing. We'd all been cautioned about the dangers of getting too close – not too short, not too long, smile, but not in a way that might seem suggestive.

The way you avoided this kind of destruction was to keep your head down. It followed that if you were prepared to put your head above the parapet then perhaps you deserved everything you got.

By controlling Britney and women like her they controlled us all, performing a stoning so relentless and public it was a shot fired into the night sky, warning us not to take another step. Anyone daring to take on the game had better learn that there are limited ways to win and every other outcome will be a loss.

Until we fully reckon with the way we were objectified and how we tortured ourselves, we will remain those girls who have been persecuted through time. Every part of our lives is connected – we are a long line stretching all the way back and propelling all the way forward.

Ageing does not happen in a vacuum to the woman who has no connection to the young girl I once was. She is deep inside me, manifested in many ways as she walked to the shops to buy a packet of chips in her white jeans and flower tank top. That girl still lives here.

And so I wanted to understand the threads that bound all those parts together, the threads that hold the key to a stage further down the road: rage.

Fire

CHAPTER 3

Rubbed in Ash:
Invisibility

THERE IS NO BLOOD test to diagnose the condition of oldness. Instead, like all the worst kinds of shonky medical procedures, it's a backyard job – a clumsy, cultural happening.

This is how it all began. It was late in the afternoon – I remember it so clearly. The uneven footpath. The loudness of the city. The colour of the sky. And the energy between us. Strange, really, on reflection, that it would have imprinted itself so strongly, but perhaps we all remember a time like this, the moment when you are changed. Even if you don't realise at the time that the change will have any significance.

We were heading out to see some music, I think, or maybe we were just going out to drink aimlessly at a pub. Most likely it was the latter, as that was what we mostly did in our early twenties so that we might fill the spare time we seemed to have, between work and study, before an online life would find a way to have us never feel that way again. And like many women who move in packs, we were connected to each other, possibly learnt much earlier for safety, but so practised now that we barely noticed how we could feel each other so acutely.

The city was full, and the sun was just starting to hide behind the tall buildings. There was an excitement in the air that happens at the start of spring. We approached a building site where there were men still working. As we walked towards it, I felt us change together, like the synchronised movements of a flock of birds who somehow know how to fly in perfect formation. A murmuration of women. Our backs stiffened, our heads all lifted slightly, we stopped talking. We weren't easily intimidated. We would show them.

But as we walked past them, nothing.

Nothing at all.

Silence.

We made it a safe distance away and stopped and looked at each other, confused. 'What the hell was that?' one of us said to the laughter of the others. 'Do we need to go home and get changed?' We were immediately conscious of the absurdity of our reaction. We had all understood from a young age that you shouldn't encourage that sort of attention, and you certainly didn't appreciate it. Only sluts would want that kind of thing.

But what was this? Suddenly, it seemed, and possibly in that moment, we had become invisible. I had spent all those years, since that first walk to the milk bar, being ready to be watched. Being watched felt rote; being watched lived inside me. Being looked at from the outside had become a way that I also learnt to see myself.

I saw myself through the eyes of anyone who looked me up and down, making notes or commentary. 'Your clothes are dirty,' my parents would say as I tried to sneak out the back door in a stained t-shirt and a pair of ripped jeans.

I thought I was always going to be looked at. But on that day, it ended abruptly. There was a distinct moment when the street fell silent. Suddenly, no one called to me anymore. Not from a truck or a shop. No one tooted as they drove past. No one tried to draw my eyes to them so they could mouth something shocking.

I wanted to understand how it happened so quickly. How we found ourselves so swiftly cut from the picture and shifted to the outer. Was the fire that brought the first sign of life, the site for the creation of us as young girls, also the fire that would reduce us to ash?

When I first noticed that the attention had shifted, I would make a point of sharing notes about when it had randomly emerged again. 'Score. I was tooted today on my way to work.' A high five would be the response. There was laughter at first as we recognised that we had suddenly been discarded and that we had all seemingly relied upon it in one way or another. It was almost a secret absurdity that we shared having spent so long rolling our eyes and performing disgust at the attention. Now it was gone, what did that mean?

Surely, I quietly believed, my suddenly not being interesting to them was only a momentary aberration. But it seemed I had been transformed with a blade that cut swiftly and without any discussion. The fire that had been so bright was now a barely glowing pile of ash and embers.

At the same time, I was giddy with the freedom. It felt as if I had been given leave from national service. I was filled with a rush of excitement that I was no longer needed for the job I had been lumped with for all those years. The job of decoy, the body that would walk around the streets to keep the hunger at bay. To ensure that everyone knew it was there if it needed to be taken.

And when suddenly it seemed no one was looking at me anymore, I felt like it was possible to creep out of my hiding place and begin to wonder just exactly who I was.

We had long moaned about the attention and told ourselves it was an insult to who we really were. It would have been shameful to admit that I felt a rush of validation with it or relief that we were attractive to the glaring force of male power.

Was the fire that was once full of promise and warmth the fire that would destroy me? Was this the same fire that I had sensed as a girl, that fed without regard for life and ran wild through any fuel source with a hunger that would kill anything in its way?

How stupid we must have been, we realised, to be so convinced by the attention we received as young girls. We believed there might be some real value for us – we foolishly believed we were new and not, as we were beginning to understand, part of a long continuum of all the women who had walked before us. 'Stupid girl,' I heard the wind spit. 'Stupid, stupid girl.'

It was the beginning of the end. I was being forgotten, not seen any longer for the life force that pulsed through my body. Dried out from the heat that erupted upon my skin.

* * *

When we are removed from the landscape and looked over – looked through – there is an incredible smarting to the erasure. A visceral rage. We have done our service in this world, keeping the baying wolves placid, scratching around in the dirt to build our homes and feed our children, and done so while being ridiculed for our form. It is not our desire for youth, as we have been told; rather, it is rage at the callousness of being discarded now that we are no longer desirable to feast upon.

To be ejected without a parting gift or engraved pen for our years of service is humiliating. We did everything you wanted of us, didn't we? We didn't complain. Well, not much. And if we did, we knew you'd find a way to destroy us, so we shut up quick. We learnt how you needed us to be. Was it that we missed a spot? We can go over it again if that will help.

The reason we were catcalled when we were as young as eleven exists for the same reasoning we are not catcalled anymore: conquest. As we age, we no longer represent a conquest to be won. We have been colonised and corrupted, and now it feels that the mission is about burning down our villages so there is no proof that they ever stormed our homes. We are disappeared into the night.

It feels as if your skin has become translucent, see-through, like a ghost. Or like a piece of fabric once heavy and immutable that is now fraying and thin. When it first happens you want to scream, 'I'm here. Can't you see me?'

For all those years, walking so carefully with my eyes downcast so as not to rock the boat or cause anyone to be mad, it seemed as if this might be who I would always be. So interconnected was I to the idea of being judged that it was like it had become a part of who I was. I thought I would always find myself travelling the world as the object of some sort of attention – certainly not often good attention, but seen and judged at least. But I soon realised, just as I had been warned, that there is a time when you are not needed for the game anymore.

Those calls from the street, from the fat men with broken teeth, were now not for me. Those calls were happening to a different fourteen-year-old girl who was walking to the shops to buy chips. And while I still felt like her and that nothing much had changed inside me, I had been made old – or, at least, not young.

Each of the ways we are changed and objectified happens like a magic trick. Just as you were transformed by the eyes that hungered for you when you were young into something for them to feast upon, so too now you are changed as their object. But this time you are taught that you are no longer wanted.

No one needs to call out to that.

And while I was dealing with this enforced invisibility and trying to understand how this had rendered me see-through in places where I might have once had a voice, I was reminded by trans advocate Yves Rees that invisibility is a privilege some women are unable to access. While the trans community has been advocating for visibility and to have their experience as women included in the conversation, it is also important to note that the invisibility that cis women experience is a privilege not always afforded to trans women.

As Erique Zhang reflects in their article 'The radical act of invisibility on Trans Day of Visibility', 'Now, as an openly trans person, I have become hypervigilant to combat my hypervisibility. When I go outside, I am keenly aware of every passing gaze. I'm constantly anticipating being recognized as trans. I try to draw as little attention to myself as possible when I'm in public because I know that the more people look at me, the higher my risk of being attacked.'[1]

* * *

Unlike changes in the self that were undertaken when we were young, when, like caterpillars, we would curl up in a cocoon to transform while our hearts beat with hope for what might emerge, there is no heady anticipation for how you withdraw and start the journey of older age. The withdrawal seems like it might be a loss rather than the beginning of something new. To begin with, this disappearance felt like it was about an absence. A space that had become suddenly empty.

I had heard, in whispers from other women, that most of us will eventually disappear. Unlike the transition from girl to woman, moving into an older body is about the act of disrobing, undressing from the identity we had spent our lifetimes forming. This time is not about the bright dresses that we found to wear, or the way we learnt to apply paint to our lips. This time is about removing a layer of skin so that you are rubbed raw in readiness to start the process of beginning again.

It was hard for me to imagine that I was suddenly someone else in their eyes. How was it that I would need to form again? To understand myself differently somehow? To cast a new mould of myself, I guess, in the same fire that cast me in the beginning? Was I the same, deep down in my organic matter? Or was I now an entirely new person?

As I moved into this older form, I realised there was no reference for how I was to carefully lower my garments so that I might travel the rest of the journey without the cover of cloth. How do you prepare to become invisible? To seep into the soil like water and disappear?

In *The Key of Solomon the King*, a book of spells written during the Renaissance and falsely attributed to the biblical King Solomon, a method of how to 'render oneself invisible' is shared. The process is fairly clear but involves killing a frog, so not wholly endorsed here. First, construct a human form made of yellow wax in the month of January and in the day and hour of Saturn. Then, above the crown and the skull of the wax figurine and also upon a small strip of skin of a dead frog or a toad, etch with a needle, characters that look like this:

$$\text{C-H-}\mathbf{3}\mathbf{8}\mathbf{+}$$

Then suspend the figure by one of your hairs from the vault of a cavern at the hour of midnight. Waft the figure with incense and call some spirits to you:

METATRON, MELEKH, BEROTH, NOTH, VENIBBETH, MACH, and all ye, I conjure thee, O Figure of wax, by the Living God, that by the virtue of these Characters and words, thou render me invisible, wherever I may bear thee with me. Amen.[2]

Bury the figurine in a wooden box until you need to become invisible. When you seek invisibility, simply dig up the box and say, 'Come unto me and never quit me wherever I shall go' until you're finished spying or hiding, or whatever it is you need to be invisible for. Just return the box to the same spot when you're done.

In the modern era, the magic of disappearance can be conjured in a much simpler way; that is, for some woman, you simply need to age. And just like that, under any moon at all, you will disappear. And with this newfound power, you can walk around a busy city street and be entirely unseen.

The first moments happen simply. You're standing at the counter at the baker or waiting to buy a beer at the bar, and what once would have been immediate recognition from the person serving you suddenly changes. You're second or third. They just didn't see you standing there. 'Is it happening?' I started to wonder.

There are many ways that I have attempted to bargain with this loss. Trying in some way to try to halt the enforcement of this change, begging for a reprieve. But before we find ways to deny it, ageing is about that initial smarting. The slap across the face that has you confused and looking around in a panic to discover if anyone else saw it and is as indignant as you.

At first, becoming older and invisible feels like the liberation you have always hungered for. The chains that have hung around your legs and arms drop to the dirt and you feel you may float to the ceiling. You are finally free. They nudge at your back, pushing you towards the door. 'Go on then,' they say, barely looking at you. But you don't move because this is all that you've known. Where would you go, anyway?

There was a fizz inside me knowing that I could now leave the house with pyjamas on and more likely affirm my own stereotype than disrupt it. Author Cate Kennedy recently remarked at a function, 'I make sure there is a whole lot going on with my outfits, so no one can put a finger on exactly what's gone wrong.'

Heading into this sphere of age and knowing that I'm no longer of interest to this hungry world was initially exciting. But it becomes clear that when you're given your pass, you need to know what you will do. It's not as if they are telling you that there is a better world waiting for you on the other side, it's just that no one needs anything from you in this one anymore. 'Could you please vacate the room? We have a new resident wanting to check in.'

It's all made very clear to us – there will be no subsidy. No help. No welfare payment for service to the community. Yes, you're free, but if you get thirsty out there, you'll have to find your own water, your own food. 'We can't help everyone,' they say.

This is not a casual omission from the landscape.

This is erasure.

Fire

CHAPTER 4

Fire Inside: The Mother

WHEN I WAS YOUNG, there was a burning inside me. A fire. A hunger that was raw and otherworldly. It sat just below words and ached in my bones. I would find out soon enough that it was a yearning for a child, a yearning so strong that I could feel it in my teeth and would grind my jaws together at night to find some relief.

Tellus Mater, or Terra Mater, was the ancient Roman goddess known as the earth mother. She was most often seen rising from a hole in the ground. Her Greek counterpart is Gaia. In similar imagery, Gaia is also seen rising partially from the earth or reclining on it.[1]

Isis, the ancient Egyptian mother, symbolises magic, marriage, fertility and medicine. She is depicted as both a goddess and a human and inspired fervent devotion from people throughout Egypt and Europe. There is speculation that she was an early inspiration for the Christian symbol of motherhood, the Virgin Mary.[2]

One thing all these figures have in common is their absolute power – the birther is the only portal to this world. And while we need them for this access, for our heirs to take their rightful place, we must ensure their safety. We must balance our desire to kill them with our need to protect them for this task.

* * *

The mother is a redemption story, positioned as selfless and nurturing, the life spring of the universe. And while she is bountiful and bursting with fertility, the world has a great interest in protecting her.

We are taught that those alluring bodies that invite colonisation can be saved if they engage in a sanctified relationship and birth children. They have the opportunity to save themselves from sexual destruction if they transform into a mother.

Being regarded as sacred is transitional and conditional. On either side of the mother image sits the maiden and the crone, two women who are dangerous. The mother ideal sits perfectly between this symmetry, momentarily holding this destruction at bay. The mother is portrayed as the holy portal to this world and therefore it's a time when a woman must be protected. It is the most holy of all because it is held separate from any relationship to desirability. For this precise time in her life, at least, the woman is considered sacred. But of course, only if she can and will birth.

It was my destiny, I was taught, to become a mother. As a child, I had many baby dolls thrust into my hands that I could hold and practise with. I was taught that being a girl would mean I would become a nurturer. Biology and health classes are geared towards teaching that the people with female physiology are, for a period of their lives, in grave danger of becoming pregnant, and then later in grave danger of not becoming pregnant, and then later still, barren.

This body belongs to everyone. Pregnant people are often touched by strangers, the roundness of their bellies stroked and held without permission. Pregnant bodies are seen as public space because they enact a public role, one that is being done for king and country. Hands reach out to touch but it is not sexualised; rather, this body is worshipped, and the new life that it holds within is somehow the property of this post-industrialised world. As if a woman was always just here for the service of childbearing.

Women are told that our service is not only to our families, our partners and our parents but also to our countries. Many politicians have uttered a version of the famous words of treasurer Peter Costello, who in 2002 implored the women of Australia to 'have one for mum, one for dad and one for the country'.[3] Population growth as economic imperative.

In this modern capitalist model we are birthing consumers and workers, and thus, the mother is the most holy of the trinity. The most necessary. The most linked to her utility. What are we here for if not to birth children?

To be truly sacred, though, there are conditions, and the woman cannot take a wrong step. She must play this role perfectly.

* * *

Being a woman is so intrinsically linked to being a mother that the two states are often treated as one. 'How many children do you have?' is a question women are often asked, the assumption so deeply embedded into the expectation of her that it's not *if* but how many. And mothering is spoken about in such exclusive ways, suggesting women who are not mothers have perhaps missed out on some vital ingredient of being a woman.

Many women do not have bodies that can become pregnant or can birth. For mine, sickness threatened that my body would not perform the task I had been assured it would. Illness had become such a large part of my life and identity when I was diagnosed with Crohn's disease in my early twenties that it consumed me and my thoughts of myself. After years of being sick, by the time they stamped my form with a diagnosis, I couldn't eat and was barely able to walk. 'I am the sickness,' I would whisper.

What I didn't realise when I was young and imagining my life as a mother was that I would bring myself to this role, and that I was literally none of the things I had believed a mother was. I had been so constructed to see the mother as an entity beyond our individual personalities that I saw myself embodying only the 'idea' of the mother.

Illness shifted my identity so strikingly that I suffered a death with it. Many deaths, in fact. Death to the dreams I had for the old body that I for so long believed was my birthright. I underwent a seismic shift in the dreams that I knew were no longer possible.

For years, I made a deep trail between my share house and the hospital. And soon, as illness continued to make an attack on my body, I lost hope that I would, that it would, ever hold a child. I tried to shut down any desire for it as the wanting was too painful. I became tired with the idea of becoming pregnant. If it wasn't for me, I wasn't interested in holding out hope for it.

The medication I was on also played havoc with the 'me' in the mirror. I was inflated and covered in pimples. I had lost hair. It felt like I was dripping in oil and sadness. I hated looking at myself. But the only way to keep the pain from consuming me whole was to outright reject these desires. 'They are not for you,' I would sternly whisper. 'You haven't lost anything that wasn't intended for you. Do not mourn this life, it was not meant for you to live.'

Just as I had done when my body oozed pus out of perianal abscesses into pads in my underpants, I decided that I no longer needed to be attractive in the world, or to expect that this ill body would give me a child. 'This is not for you,' I would growl. 'How stupid that you thought it would be.'

I looked at my friends who had given birth and who were tired and undone from the experience, buried in the exhausting first years of parenting. Even still, I longed to be in their bodies. The grit of their tired skin that made them want to cry. Their eyes burning with fatigue. I wanted to feel what it was like, and I wanted to know the experience of birth. What was this transcendent pain that they all spoke about? My own pain, full of loss and 'disfiguration', had never felt like that.

Even on that day when she was discovered inside me, I was too sick to have ever believed this might be possible for someone like me. That through this body I might become pregnant. My partner and I had begun the process of looking at other options. Could we adopt? Should we concentrate on being carers and foster many, many children? We began down the path of IVF.

* * *

It was my body that first knew there was a child hidden inside and was desperately trying to tell me. In the way that our bodies must always be trying to be heard, those wordless messages shot through to every cell to announce to me that she was there. 'Wake up, child,' was what it was like. 'Surely you must feel her energy inside you? She has arrived.'

It was like my blood and my skin were screaming at me to feel that she had been there now for weeks, tucked away under all that was broken in my body. 'Trust me,' was its plea. But I had lost trust in this body long ago. I had forgotten how to feel it from the inside, as I had been taught to instead watch it from the outside. Critical of my body's every move, I had forgotten what it was like to be grounded like a tree, with my roots deep inside me.

When my body was screaming at me to notice that she was there, I had already spent much of my illness ignoring my body's painful lurch. I ignored the sounds of a baby who was moving through my blood. But eventually, on an afternoon before I was due to go to hospital the next morning for a procedure, I found out that I was pregnant.

From mourning the unlikely possibility of becoming a mother, I now found myself taking on the task of a baby housed in a broken vessel. My body was not perfect, or pure as I had long seen as the dominant representation of a pregnant body. Instead, it was unreliable and dangerous. Was this going to be my punishment for wanting something so grand and holy? I wore the trauma of this responsibility every day of the pregnancy. How could I stay well enough to bring her to earth safely? I was not the image of the mother that I had been taught to honour.

By the time I was pregnant, my disease had progressed through my system so that I needed an ileostomy bag. It was the greatest revenge on those people with hands that felt it was their place to touch my belly without request when they brushed over the bag that was hidden underneath layers of clothing. They would look at me with confusion and I would smile back. 'That's my ileostomy bag.' Then think wickedly, 'You have entered my private space – this is what you deserve.'

A woman chased me up an escalator once. I turned, expecting her to tell me I had dropped money or left something behind in a shop. Instead, she reached out and rubbed my belly. 'So beautiful,' she cooed. 'Such a beautiful thing to be pregnant.' I smiled politely, not sure exactly what my reaction should be. 'Thanks?' was all I could muster.

As with illness, a pregnant body can become pathologised if seen through the prism of a medical system that often regards it simply as a biology housing another biology. The body is gelled and probed and inserted with metal objects. And it is fundamentally othered, often divorced from the person who lives inside it. Divorced from the earth that we supposedly sit half in, half out.

Many women are traumatised by this othering, being treated as if their bodies do not have them inside. 'But this is my body,' they plead to efficient health workers, who assure them they care about this fact but sometimes deny them the autonomy to make decisions on its behalf. The trauma of being treated like you know less than someone who lives outside your body has harmed people for generations.

I experienced a form of birth trauma, although I wouldn't have described it like that at the time. I believed it was just how birth happened, the utter terror I felt when I didn't know if I could bring my children through from the other side safely. And I suffered enormously post-birth with something that felt akin to how I have heard PTSD described. The wild experience of feeling that you have come so close to your own death and the death of your child makes it seem as though recovery might be impossible. The responsibility of being a broken body. The ugliness of it all. The blackness.

And we take the trauma of birth and of not living up to the stereotype of the mother into the remainder of our lives as parents, scrutinised now for the behaviour of our children – what we feed them, if they are polite or dirty or behave strangely and climb on the furniture. And we bear the burden of these perceived failures and place them deep inside us, doing the work of the oppressor to ensure that we won't use our power for long. We must be reminded that we have likely failed and that, in truth, we are not worth much. Not really. We may be the all-powerful portal, but soon enough we are made small again – reminded that the power we may have had is just fleeting – just a moment.

* * *

I can hear her breath behind me, staged and thin. 'I told you, wait till we get home,' she whispers, trying to contain the energy that is building inside her. The child drops immediately to the floor and screams with a fever and intensity that is always surprising when it erupts from such a small body. I turn around to look at her so that she knows I get it and I'm on her side and that I've been there before, but she is too consumed by what is happening to register why I'm looking.

She returns my look with one that suggests she wants to kill me. She wants to kill us all. She hates us for seeing her like this. So I quickly look away as she pulls at his arm to try to get him up. 'I told you that you won't be getting anything today. Stand up … Stand *up!*' she yells. She looks desperate, and I can hear a grief in her voice. She is shaking. And the child continues to scream. She drops the clothes and kitchen items that she had been lining up to buy and, with everything she has, picks him up and carries him towards the door as he kicks and tries to wrestle his way out of her arms. 'No, Mummy, no!'

'You've left your other things,' a shop assistant calls after her, but we all know she's not coming back for them. Nothing is worth the public humiliation of being seen as a bad mum. That's what she's thinking – that she's a bad mum. Why else would her kid be doing this to her?

'Failed mother' is a belief seething inside so many who become one. 'Mother's guilt' is a ubiquitous term for a person who has fallen short of the image they have seen since they themselves were a child. The mother image is serene – giving without complaint. Joyful at the prospect of servicing their needs last. They are the eternal giver, the one who sacrifices. The one who should be fed last but who feeds others well. The mother is harried and beautiful.

Mother's guilt can come about by the sheer intensity of the role of parenting. That intensity is often housed in the most banal setting and occupied by the most boring of jobs. Parental burnout can explain the deep feelings of shame and inadequacy that are often experienced by parents and can largely be attributed to cultural influences. Countries that place a higher value on individualism were more likely to have parents who would burn out.[4]

Parents are now expected to be more attentive, more focused on their children than ever before. There has been a giant shift in the manner in which parents are perceived compared to the past – what was considered good parenting fifty years ago would be perceived as neglectful now. There is an expectation that parents are responsible to minimise any potential risks while simultaneously ensuring successful physical, intellectual, social and emotional development. Anything less than highly efficient and strategic parenting that will harness the best of their young offspring is sold as neglectful. No longer do we question needs vs. wants of our children; instead, every advantage is essential and expected to be sought by a good parent.[5]

We are told how we can be good mothers. How we will serve the role well. We are given advice. We are policed for the food we eat, whether the cheese is too soft or the coffee unnecessary. We believe that if we love our children, a good mother will sacrifice. And we will be pleased to work hard for our families because the gift we have been given is this life-giving power. To misuse it or take it for granted or not pay its debt is sacrilege.

And when the children arrive, we must adore playdough. And wrap them in blankets and sing them lullabies and read them enough books to ensure they will be given a scholarship to a good high school and teach them Spanish and order them the right educational toys so they can start to build necessary fine and gross motor skills.

In recent history, the sense of failure has been exacerbated by the prevalence of mummy (mommy) as an industry. The rise of mummy bloggers, who share their experience of motherhood online through blogs and social media, have made the mother image aspirational. This is an intense period of scrutiny for a woman: how your body copes with the demands of birth, how well it returns to its former size and elasticity, how beautiful you look, how devoted you are to your children.

But it's also unsurprising how denigrated the idea of a mother writing about her experience is and the way they are referred to as mummies, as if it is an extension of the vacuous behaviours of the teenagers they once were. But there is no denying how suffocating the promulgation of 'mummy' is to many women. I was so harassed by the idea of being a mummy, so suffocated by the perception that I had suddenly become only one identity, that I refused to go to the assigned parenting group after the birth of my first child. Instead, I sent my husband.

* * *

Some people give birth in bodies that do not identify as women, and with imagery that is all about women and birth, and a strong cultural idea that birth is only done by women, it can be extremely traumatic for people who give birth who identify outside this gendered concept.

Steph had felt alien in the body that they had been born into. So confused were they with the changes that took place as a twelve-year-old, when they started to develop into a teenager, that they stopped eating. The dissonance of living with female biology when you did not feel like a girl was unbearable, they explained; it was heartbreaking. But Steph grew up in a cultural time when identities beyond a binary were not spoken about so much. It certainly wasn't something that the people around them knew about, or that Steph knew how to convey to anyone. So, instead, Steph stopped eating, a reaction from somewhere beyond their consciousness or decision making so that they might stop growing the body that didn't feel like it belonged to them. This was in the hope it might stop the whirring confusion of what they were turning into, something that didn't fit the picture they had of themselves in their mind's eye.

In their mid-thirties, they are just starting their pronoun adventure: 'I think most people who know me properly understand the energy of me, but I can communicate for myself so much better now. The power of the evolving language is amazing and it's nice when someone clues into it and clocks you. I think it's about broadening the understanding of what humans can be and are. As my daughter puts it, quite plainly and clearly, "Some people are in the middle." Through the development of the language, I now see how many people have had or are having the same feelings as me that would have been invaluable to me as an adolescent when I felt totally alone.'

They had become a parent a couple of years ago when their partner birthed their first child, but when they tried for a sibling, it became clear that Steph may need to carry if they wanted a second child. The idea of their body growing in this way was difficult to accept at first. 'Yeah, it's been absolutely surreal.' Steph laughs, indicating the utter ridiculousness of it all, that their body might do this. 'But we were lucky to have two uteruses to work with, and I eventually thought, you know what? I can try, and yes, I am flying far, far above myself in another brain realm – but I'm doing it! My partner has been amazing, often catching my thoughts or reactions before I do, and I've built a scaffolding of support. I feel lucky. And this process has also taught me a lot; it's given me the confidence to explain myself as I am.'[6]

We had spoken years before about there being no way possible for them to think about their body in this way. 'I definitely couldn't do it,' they'd said then, the idea too foreign to conceive of. 'In figuring it out, I knew I'd have to have a caesarean because it was the way I could get my head around doing it. In controlling some of the factors, and in keeping the continuity of care – that has been really important to help with communicating the situation. I've been lucky to have found a trans-friendly healthcare worker in the system. Without our midwife Jess advocating for me, truly going into bat for me, I would not have been able to do this, and for them I am truly grateful.'

* * *

First Nations women and families had their babies stolen. Almost quaintly, we now refer to an entire generation of people who were forcibly removed from their families as the 'Stolen Generation', as if they are simply a mass of people in our history rather than the detailed names and experiences that this Stolen Generation represents. But the numbers are multiplied by the generational trauma that such forcible removals have had on family groups since. The *Bringing Them Home* report estimated that somewhere between one in ten and one in three children were removed from families and communities between 1910 and 1970.

Children were forcibly removed and placed in institutions, fostered or adopted out to non-Indigenous families because white Australia and its inherent racist systems and structures didn't want to believe that Aboriginal mothers or families could care for their own children. They were robbed of their culture, language and love. A catastrophic theft that has impacted multiple generations of First Nations families. 'Good mothers', these white post-colonial powers must have believed, were not Aboriginal mothers. They simply couldn't be. And, by extension, good people could not be born from these Aboriginal bodies. Therefore, it made sense that they would need to be saved, and entire institutions and systems would be built on this racism.

The impact of this forced removal, and the racism and violence on which it was founded, is felt keenly generations on. In Australia, intergenerational trauma predominantly affects First Nations people – the children, grandchildren and future children of the Stolen Generation.

Lois Peeler AM, Yorta Yorta woman, activist and educator, sees the trauma of forced removal impacting families for generations. At Worawa Aboriginal College, a boarding school for girls in Healesville, Victoria where she is Principal, Peeler runs a program called 'Pathways to Womanhood'. 'So that's about guiding young girls in ways that perhaps they haven't had the opportunity to learn from, the mothers and the aunties, and the nanas in their community, because they might have been in the Stolen Generation.'[7,8]

* * *

For some, pregnancy can be one of the most dangerous times in their life. 'Among women who were pregnant at some time during a relationship and experienced violence with their most recent violent partner or their current partner, 54% and 22%

respectively reported that they were pregnant at the time of the violence and 25% and 13% reported that violence occurred for the first time during pregnancy (ABS 2013).'[9]

Intimate partner violence and domestic violence during a pregnancy increases the risk three-fold of being a victim of an attempted/completed murder for women who are abused during pregnancy than among those who are not.[10]

If a woman has somehow fallen, and it's easy to fall, she becomes one of the darkest versions of this archetype. Sluts can find themselves getting 'knocked up' if they aren't careful. These are not the women who deserve the same kind of treatment as married women. These are not the women we think of when we imagine the sacred.

The forced removal of newborn babies from unwed mothers by institutions was considered the best solution to an adoption crisis in Australia when it began in the 1950s. It also served to save children from their 'illegitimacy' after being born by 'sexual deviants' who were deemed 'unfit' to parent. As described by human rights activist and academic Christine Cole in a *Vice* article in 2017, 'I was pushed back onto the bed by three nurses. The pillow was placed back on my chest and the midwife at the end of the bed said, "This has got nothing to do with you ..." We were considered to have gotten pregnant because we were morally and mentally inferior – therefore, not mentally stable to bring up a child.'[11] It is estimated that there were potentially 250,000 forced adoptions across Australia from the 1950s to the 1980s.[12]

For the women who know they don't want children, it is a constant experience of explaining why. Of finding reasons that satisfy those who pretend to be making thoughtful enquiries about your life. But really, of what interest is this to anyone else? Except that we have been told since we were children ourselves that this is what a woman does. A woman births.

If you are in a steady relationship, or if you've just got married, expect that question regularly. If you are a woman entering her thirties, regardless of your partner status, expect that question with an added head tilt to show a deep understanding of the pain you might be feeling.

There is a time in your life when it seems that you are required to reveal if you intend to use your body for its capacity to birth. The sly looks from older women who sidle up to you at the family party and edge around the question. 'Are you enjoying work?' they might ask at first. Then perhaps they might go in, straight and hard. 'Are you thinking of a family?'

How are you expected to explain to someone that you don't want to have a baby? Not now, not ever. Well-meaning friends will ask, 'Are you sure?' Because, of course, this will be the greatest regret of your life, they tell you with their sad eyes.

* * *

Carrie had been unwell for some time. Her unrelenting fatigue and bloating had made it hard for her to leave the house on the weekends. She was just scraping her way through the work week, desperate to find her way to bed at the end of every day. It took the health profession a long time to diagnose her. For most of the time when seeking help she was met with a raised eyebrow and a 'perhaps you need to see a psychologist' response. Finally, she began to get some answers. She had a heart condition that had led to chronic fatigue, and there was growing speculation that she had entered early menopause.

Heading into her middle thirties and recently married, Carrie knew she was going to be asked about children. In fact, she knew she had better be prepared to find a way to navigate the endless enquiries that would come from family and friends. What she didn't expect was to be taken aside by her boss at her accounting firm and asked explicitly if she had plans to have children.

'Well, no,' she stammered. 'We don't plan to have children, but I'm not sure what that has to do with ...' Her boss was quick to reassure her it was just a friendly chat. 'We'd love to see you grow in this company no matter what you decide to do. But if we're thinking about the short term, of course, I'm just interested in finding out what you're planning. We might have a bigger role here for you.'

It wasn't just work and her family – the questions about her body came from everywhere. Due to her bloating condition she would sometimes wear looser fitting tops. One night, at a party, an older man approached her and her partner and with a wink offered his congratulations. Carrie's partner assumed he must have heard something about them getting married. 'Thanks, yeah, we got married a year ago.'

But Carrie knew his assessment was about her body. 'I'm not pregnant,' she said, smiling, hoping this wasn't going to end up being awkward. Embarrassed, he tried to cover it up by saying, 'Oh, then you're just fat, I guess. How was I to know?'

She felt an explicit question around her womanhood was often present in these exchanges, that somehow she must have done something to be in a position of not wanting a baby. 'What do I tell people?' she asked me one afternoon, trying to find a way to avoid the constant feelings of inadequacy. 'How do I tell people that I just don't want to do it? No one believes that it's possible that I don't want to have a baby.' She had begun to question herself: 'Am I selfish? Is there something wrong with me that I don't want a child?'

* * *

Our experience of feeling childless can happen later in our lives when the eternity of time spent as mothers comes to an end. We parent our children in a myriad of ways, feeding them, dressing them and holding them through the night, right up until they are finishing school and then finding their way through the world as people in their own right. All the noise, the mess, every part of the process that you prayed would one day get easier is suddenly gone.

The game of parenting is such that the ultimate aim is to become obsolete. Of course, you will always have an important place in the lives of your children, but your role as a parent – one who keeps them safe, feeds them, guides them, clothes them, is vital for their survival – comes to an end.

For some women, the mother identity is a difficult one to relinquish. Many women are lost without the deep sense of meaning and purpose that mothering gave their lives. 'Empty nest syndrome', while not an official medical diagnosis, is attributed to parents who experience deep sadness, depression, a crisis of identity and even symptoms of grief when their children finally leave the family home.

'She left when she was twenty-two,' Marnie tells me, 'and I fell into a depression. For months I couldn't get out of bed.' Marnie had loved being a mother – the labour, the emotional role that she played in her daughter's life, the closeness, seeing her grow up and become a wonderful adult. And when she left,

Marnie didn't know what to do with herself. 'I didn't want to give her up. I wanted to cook for her, to clean, to support her – I didn't know what to do without her. She's been such a wonderful part of my life.'

When my partner and I had our first child, we once lay awake in bed in the middle of the night, alert with a white fear. Cold blood moved through me. A dryness in my mouth. 'Why did we think we could do this?' I said, knowing he would understand what I meant. 'Why weren't we satisfied with what we had? Now we've been given this gold, and for the rest of our lives we are charged with keeping it safe. I don't think I can do this,' I whispered. He laughed. 'One hundred per cent agree. What were we thinking?'

I slid back down with only my eyes protruding from the sheets. This is how I've slept since.

Fire

CHAPTER 5

Burnt at the Stake: The Witch

ONCE A YEAR WE would have our foreheads rubbed with ash. The priest with his thick thumbs would mark us with a black cross, one by one, to remind us of our death and that we were sinners. I loved this ritual simply because it broke the monotony of the school day. We would file down to the back of the school grounds, where the church, which loomed so large on our small landscape, was all we could see. It blocked the skyline and the view onto the street. And it bore down on me, making it feel like it might be my everything.

I was only eight. I ran my fingers up and down the cross on my forehead. Marked. Reminded that we had been burnt before. Destroyed by fire so that we were left as only black dust. A dirty mark.

* * *

I sat in stunned silence as our Year 2 teacher, Mrs Halge, read us the story of Hansel and Gretel. I shared in the visceral fear Hansel and Gretel must have felt when they were tricked by the witch and her gingerbread house, so she could eat them. How cunning that witch had been to coax the children and then lock them up, fattening up Hansel until his large, juicy body could be devoured by her, limb by limb. 'Why would she do that?' I wondered in shock.

In the early versions of the story, it was their mother who initially abandons Hansel and Gretel, and then in later versions that woman becomes the wicked stepmother.[1] Our mythology is riddled with the bad version of mother. The relationship between the witch and the evil stepmother is often interchangeable. That women might ruin or wish to harm children simmers below the surface of our concept of these types of mothers and draws a direct relationship between a woman's body and her ability to be a good person.

At the heart of our fear of witches was that their treachery was merciless and their desire to destroy seemingly unquenchable. We feared them because their powers were not of this world. Old witches were especially dangerous because they'd been cast out and had nothing left to lose.

Oldness is so despised that there is an entitlement to, in turn, despise the women who inhabit these ageing bodies. Women are a commodity of both sex and servitude, and as we age, we become unnecessary for both. And then we are carefully erased, buried deep beneath the human psyche, mocked and condescended to.

Beyond thin character portraits seen only sometimes in

film, often built on tropes and stereotypes, old women have largely been written out of existence. But it's more than being written out. It's more than suddenly finding that your skin is see-through. There is an active intent to turn our eyes away from this old woman. To deliberately see through her. To make sure she knows that she is only as good as we allow her to be. If we can unsee her, she has no power over us.

* * *

I realised that ageing was going to be forced upon me as a reflection of how useful I was now perceived to be. How fast I was. How at odds I suddenly felt about the world around me. How worthwhile I felt. How attractive. How fit. How well I had done in my career. Had I mothered? If so, how well were my children coping in the world?

It felt almost impossible to remove my identity from how the world needed me. The idea that ageing is related to our utility was not something I had previously understood properly. I had seen *Thomas the Tank Engine* and realised that old engines would be taken to the scrap heap. But I hadn't realised this was likely an allegory written to warn old people of what was to come.

While I worked hard to convince myself that this was what I had wanted – that I wanted to age and seep into the earth – the truth was I had been forced into this change and into the idea of what being old was all about. I was determined to decree that I had control over it somehow, that I was excited about getting older, about leaving my youth behind. That I had no problems with moving into a new stage of life. But the truth was something else altogether.

Just as I had been forced to participate in the treatment of my past forms – the girl, the young woman, the mother – now my personhood was being dictated to me as a sudden removal from the landscape. It was the beginning of not being needed. At least, not in the ways I had been needed in the past.

With these sorts of changes, this kind of cultural shaping, there isn't a great deal of negotiation that takes place. I wasn't given much warning of when I would become old. Or at least when I would be 'not young' anymore.

One day, simply, you are different in their eyes. The old woman you have always regarded with your own set of suspicions has, without warning, started the process of morphing into your form. 'Oh,' you scoff, 'I'm not old. Surely this is a mistake.'

* * *

The witch is an all-powerful woman who manipulates the world around her. She is depicted largely as gathering victims through spells and dark crafts with the aim to destroy them. And her hunger is insatiable as she goes about destroying the most valuable: young women, children of other women, unsuspecting men or anyone who dares stand in her crosshairs.

The old woman in mythology is withered. The fire has dried her skin so that now it hangs lifeless and loose. She is bereft of the lifegiving pool of liquid that once flowed through her. We see her as angry and vengeful, and she is often depicted as plotting a way to return to the form of the maiden. In nursery rhymes, the old lady tricks young girls so she can steal their young lives to be hers to live again.

Witch hunts dating back to and beyond the most infamous in Salem, Massachusetts, in 1692 show us a horrifying history into the views that were held about women and their capacity for evil. It was believed women, weaker than men in all respects, could be easily corrupted by the devil. We knew these women who were lured by the dark forces were the transgressive women, women who threatened power, women who sat outside the margins of society and women who were simply unpleasant.

What has changed?

Women who challenge the power elite, who step outside the agreed path, who enjoy a sexual identity that doesn't conform, who flout the rules, who expect sexual autonomy without violence, who tell the secrets of what happens behind those doors of power – those women will be destroyed like the women before them.

Or at least an attempt will be made on their lives.

Sarah Good was one of the first women to be accused of witchcraft during the Salem witch trials. These words have come from the ink of her pen from over three hundred years ago, but they very well might have been written today:

> We [Sarah and her second husband] lost our few acres,
> so that to live at all we had to beg. But I would not be
> servile, as a proper beggar must. I had my pride, and it
> was rubbed raw daily, until the neighbours felt that I was
> not humble, not grateful enough for their bounty. They
> construed my mumbling as curses, and perhaps they were
> right. How could I be unresentful, seeing others flourish
> who were no more deserving than I?[2]

Sarah's father was a wealthy inn owner who died by suicide when she was just seventeen years old. She would have been left part of his estate except that her mother's new husband took the bulk of the inheritance and left Sarah and her sisters with virtually nothing. Sarah's first husband died, leaving her and her next husband in debt, which ultimately meant that their home and land was taken from them. By the beginning of the witch trials, Sarah was homeless.

During her trial, those who accused Sarah of witchcraft said that she was likely envious of them. It was in February 1692 that Sarah Good was officially accused of witchcraft after two girls, Abigail Williams and Betty Parris, began behaving strangely and having fits. When questioned by adults about who was causing these fits – 'Who is it that bewitches you?' – the girls eventually accused three women: Sarah Good, Tituba, a slave, and Sarah Osborne.[3]

Although Sarah Good was likely in her late thirties when she was hanged, having just given birth to a child who died soon after and with another child who was around four and half years of age, she is depicted through historical accounts and literary references as being old. She appears as a woman who inhabited the fringes, she was described as offensive and aged, in a culture that repudiated those who were old, vulnerable and weak.[4]

Sarah Good was killed for being angry. She was killed for being unpleasant around town. For not being grateful. For challenging how a 'good' woman should behave. Good's own husband, William, told the court that he felt his wife was a witch because of her 'bad carriage to him', that he didn't like the way she treated him as his wife.

When she was preparing to be hanged, she was asked by the reverend officiating whether she was prepared to admit her guilt to save her soul. Instead of confessing, she is famously said to have screamed, 'You are a liar! I'm no more a witch than you are a wizard. If you take away my life, God will give you blood to drink.'[5] She was hanged on 19 July 1692. It is said, although difficult to verify and largely believed to be fiction, that Reverend Noyes suffered an internal haemorrhage and died choking on his own blood.[6]

* * *

Stories like Sarah Good's have been told over and over again. The thin line that travels the hundreds of years from her story to ours speaks in the same tongue. Now older women who find themselves in the hallways of power – in places they were never meant to be – are the ones who are punished. We despise them and mock them when they speak their mind or are seen to be unpleasant to those who disagree with them.

Julia Gillard, former Australian Prime Minister and the first woman to take that office, in 2010, was subjected to sexist trolling from the mainstream media, the opposition party and sectors of the public. Those who couldn't conceive of a woman taking a seat in the highest office in the country knew that the association with the witch archetype was easily made. The comparison was an easy way to explain to the public en masse that what we were dealing with was dangerous.

The message was clear: we should be sceptical of the motives of women who find their way to power like this. How did she get there? Surely not on merit. Something else must be at play. Who had she tricked or hurt to win like this? And for women like Julia Gillard who were childless, she was the type they were the most suspicious of. Women like that, we are taught, would be ruthless in their wrath. Imagine giving up motherhood for – what? A career?

They knew it would be easy to use her sex against her. To rally her ancestors to do the work for them. The then Opposition Leader, Tony Abbott, proudly stood in front of a sign reading 'ditch the witch' held by protesters outside Parliament House and allowed press photos to be taken with an assumed endorsement of the language. Other signs that crowded the frame were 'Bob Brown's bitch', referring to the then leader of the Australian Greens party. Years later, Julia Gillard wondered publicly why this blatant sexist behaviour did not end the career of Tony Abbott. Instead, far from ending it, he became the next Prime Minister of Australia.[7]

Weaponising the witch archetype is not unique to Australian politics. Hillary Clinton also endured it in 2016 during her presidential election campaign for the Democrats against Republican Donald Trump. Images of Hillary Clinton were doctored to depict her 'wearing a black hat and riding a broom, or else cackling with green skin. Her opponents named her the Wicked Witch of the Left.'[8]

In Christian mythology, this transgression begins with Eve. Said to be the first human ally of Satan, being female is what is understood to have made her susceptible to corruption. According to many historic texts, women have always been more susceptible to evil, our weakened state allowing us to be used in ways men are able to resist. So engrained are these concepts of women that it is our automatic assumption. How did they get to where they are? Did they use their bodies? Did they trick the men around them? And now, how do we destroy them?

Old women have bodies that scare little children. Their bodies are a warning to anyone young enough to heed it: watch it, you don't want to become like them. Women are compelled to comply as young girls, but importantly we find that we must also comply as old women. Those who don't, those who wish to raise their voices against the din, are easily disposed of.

The broomstick is one of the essential tools of the witch. In its domestic life, the broomstick is an emblem of being bound to the home, a symbol of servitude. But the witch conjures the broomstick instead as power. The broomstick is flight and freedom. She is a conjurer of greatness by using the power of the everyday world that surrounds her.

There is some evidence that the broomstick imagery is based in a fantasy even more incredible. During the Middle Ages it was thought that brews and ointments or salves were used for witchcraft and sorcery and 'somewhere along the line, the observation was made that the hallucinogenic compounds, hyoscine in particular – also known as scopolamine – could be absorbed through sweat glands in the armpit or via the mucus membranes of the rectum or vaginal area'.[9]

* * *

Growing up listening to tales of witches who would eat us for dinner, it was always older teachers we would think of in this way. 'Stupid old witch,' my friend spat under his breath when he had been told by a teacher that she was going to fail him that year. Her grey hair and leathery skin made her seem rottener than perhaps she was, and I wonder now, thinking back, how old she actually was. When we were young we would think of the older people in our lives in such a monolithic way. Everyone over the age of thirty was grouped together and condemned for being out of touch.

But it was always these older women teachers whom we gave the hardest time. All of us did. And they seemed emboldened by our dislike of them. As if the more we despised them and tried to rebel against their rules and ideas, the more they took a pleasure in shortening our lead and tightening our noose. As if the victory for them came in the form of our cries of dissatisfaction. I secretly loved these women but shared a fear of them. How could we not fear them after being taught since we were babies that these old women would find pleasure in our destruction?

Women have long attempted to reclaim the witch as a symbol of power.[10] 'Show me your witches and I'll show you the way you feel about women,' writes Pam Grossman in her book *Waking the Witch: Reflections on Women, Magic and Power*. And clearly we can see how the witch has been depicted through the thousands of years that she has featured in our storytelling.[11]

The witches of our modern mythology have evolved somewhat. They are more likely to be the benefactors of their power, and their power is more often used for universal good: Samantha from *Bewitched*, Sabrina the teenage witch, and Hermione Granger from the Harry Potter books. Of course, the real women who are depicted as witches in our public lives – the ones who stand up to power, who speak the truth against the shame of secrets, who talk about sexual assault – still hold a real fear for their safety in their homes, on the streets and in their workplaces.

Do the witches teach us that we feel a sense of power as we age because we no longer need to be fearful of our burning, as we have nothing left to lose? Or that we are no longer afraid of our erasure? When age enables us to understand that this burning can be our emancipation from the cast that we were struck at birth, then maybe the fire can become our power.

We have fought to see our real witches through the frame of their power, their existence a subversion of dominant cultural norms for women with a capacity to dictate and change the world around them. Real power to conjure our future. Now known around the world as the misogyny speech, Julia Gillard eventually spoke about the sexism she believed she faced in Australian politics in a parliamentary speech on 9 October 2012, focusing her attention on the then Opposition Leader Tony Abbott:

> I will not be lectured about sexism and misogyny by this man. I will not. And the government will not be lectured about sexism and misogyny by this man. Not now, not ever.[12]

From the ashes, the dust, we can dig around and find an ember and blow hard. Blow until we see another tiny flicker of light. Of life. And from this small moment of potential, we can begin again. Rubbed raw and removed from the big story of the world and returned to the ground to begin again. What will we do now, we wonder – the world is so big and I cannot be seen. Who can I be?

ELEMENT:

Air

The Wind Cries

Air

Introduction

MY SISTER WAS BORN during the dust storm that tore through Melbourne the week before the Ash Wednesday bushfires. Tonnes of topsoil was ripped from the drought-ravaged Wimmera and Mallee earth in the north-west of Victoria. It was picked up easily, as if it had meant nothing, and blown across the skies of a city that was left in darkness. I watched from the window of my grandparents' home as the sky turned black.[1]

Kneeling on the couch in their 'good room' with one of my brothers, I watched the afternoon transform into night. I was inert and silent. It's been exactly how I've responded to uncertain danger since. I'm not good in a crisis, I don't leap to lead people through disaster. Instead, I just watch and hope that someone will know what to do. I am selfish as I try to be quiet, so the danger might pass me by, while it hunts for other victims.

It was like nothing I had ever seen. I wondered whether we might be picked up and launched into the sky and taken to another world like Dorothy when she was caught in the winds that blew through Kansas. But unlike Dorothy, as this storm bore down upon us, it didn't feel like we would land in a world full of colour and magic.

I didn't know it then but an event like this can arrive as a warning, a way to tell us to be careful. It's often not the final act but the beginning of the devastation that follows. Perhaps, if I had been older, I may have understood that it was a sign of things to come.

Melbourne stayed in darkness for what felt like hours. Later that day, my dad arrived home and told us that they'd named our new baby Clare. 'It's a simple name,' he said. 'No one can shorten it. She'll be just Clare.' She was their fourth child. What he didn't understand then is that names that can't be shortened will get lengthened. Or changed.

The first time I held her in my arms I was eight years old. I looked at her like I was looking into a mirror. Was this what I was like when I was a baby? I felt the same thirty years later when I gave birth to my son, that intense sublanguage knowing that we were simply a continuum of each other. Cyclic and connected.

* * *

When it is calm, I barely notice the wind. Not the air that fills my lungs, or the wind that lifts my hair softly and dances upon my nape so that goosebumps appear almost instantly – I barely notice any of it. But when the wind needs to be felt and seen, it has a temper like any of the other elements. Without warning, the wind will become enraged and has the power to throw our bodies around. Our hair is tossed about to make us look like the fools we are. 'Stupid girl,' it squeals.

The wind created chaos in the school grounds when we were children. Teachers knew to have extra staff on duty if it was windy. It would whip through the playground, pushing hard into our lungs to remind us that we were not supposed to live quietly. Instead we should be banging our hands hard against the railing. 'I'm here,' we should scream. 'I'm *here!*' And if we're brave enough, 'Come and get me' is what we know we should taunt the world with. The wind reminds children that they are, in fact, wild.

My grandad had taught me to lick a finger and hold it up high into the wind. Whichever side of your finger became cold was the direction the wind came from.

That day I had heard that the winds were coming. I knew it wouldn't be the time for these sorts of games, but I didn't know that the wind could sound like a freight train ramming up against all the matchstick structures we had naively built. When the air promised to be gentle, we thought we could rule the earth. But when it decided to roar, the wind reminded us that all the things we hold so dear are temporary. The buildings, the signs, the flashing lights, the houses, our lives – they would all come crashing down around our ears if the wind deemed it so.

That day, when the dust storm ripped through Melbourne, it cut power to more than 150,000 people, damaged houses, train services were forced to grind to a halt, boats were ripped from where they had been moored. It has been recorded as the most extreme dust storm ever to hit the city of Melbourne.[2]

* * *

We are reminded of the impermanence of life – a fact we often conveniently forget – when the winds come through and challenge who we think we are, rearranging things just enough that we don't remember how things used to be. Or upending everything so that it now looks upside down. And when the strength of the gusts can have you facing in the wrong direction – it changes how you see the world, how you think, how your body works and you can forget who you always thought you were.

This is perhaps the great strength of air. When you are entirely discombobulated, blown off course, it becomes an opportunity to move through the confusion and the pain of living, so that maybe, just maybe you can arrive at a place that forces you to find something of yourself again. Something more clarified and elemental, unencumbered by the flashing lights and the façade. Just the bare bones.

Midlife is the time when the 'who am I?' question is hard to answer and can lead into other difficult questions. The midlife is the time before those great epiphanies they promise will come when older age descends. For me, this middle point was a time when I felt lost, when the world around me had transformed somehow. While everything looked the same, I knew that everything had changed. Or at least I had.

And it is in this state of mind, when we are lost and disoriented, that we begin to make decisions around how we think we might like to bring forth this ageing self. Or to fight like the clappers against it. To fill our faces or diet away our midlife blubber. Mostly we behave the way we do because we are living in denial of our change, our death.

I licked my finger and pointed it towards the sky, but for this storm at least, I couldn't tell which way the wind was blowing.

Air

CHAPTER 6

The Trade Winds: Body

WHEN WE WERE KIDS there was a saying: Don't make that face, the wind might change and you'll be stuck like that forever.

I saw it out the corner of my eye. At first it was small enough for me to ignore, but soon enough it was unmistakable, unavoidable. A wobble, coming from the lower part of my upper arm. 'Over there.' I pointed. And just like that, on cue, the fatty underside of my arm, once taut and muscular, wobbled like it had a life of its own. It flapped like a turkey snood. I looked around, expecting there to be a crowd of onlookers laughing at it.

When we were young we'd call those 'tuckshop lady arms'. They belonged to the bodies of the women, mostly mothers, who would don an apron and file into the school tuckshop to feed us. We laughed at their fat old arms that wobbled when they handed out our meat pies. And when it was summer and their arms were exposed and their breasts hung low, we prayed that our bodies would never betray us like this.

I remember, too, how I longed to be held by those wrinkly, saggy arms. My neighbour Betty had them, the type you wanted to be held inside. The type that would almost suffocate you with the flesh that wrapped and held you longer than you were used to. You'd try to wriggle free, but not really, because it felt so good.

When I saw my own snood, I panicked. How long had it been there? Had I been wobbling to the amusement of children, unaware? The snood seems to appear as one of the first signs of ageing. A quick search online and you'll find references to how you can get rid of your bat wings. The emergence of my own seemed like the canary in the coalmine, sent to let me know that I'd clocked over. My skin was beginning to thin and lose its elasticity, and this was just the beginning – my body was breaking down.

I laughed when I first saw the wobble and felt a solidarity with the women I had mercilessly mocked when I was a child. Initially there was a sense of pride that I now belonged to that special group of women. But how had this turkey wobble seemingly appeared overnight? I became keenly aware of every tiny wobble the snood made and even shared it with others. 'Check it out,' I would say. 'I have tuckshop lady arms.'

And with every disparaging remark I made about my body I knew I was playing a part in the mockery I had been taught to deal out to the bodies of older women since the time when mine was young. I had learnt that the old woman's body was funny, one that you were expected to cover up and hide away under layers of clothing. You cannot believe that it might be beautiful – that was unthinkable – and certainly, you were expected to keep it from view.

At the local pools when I was eight or nine, I would be fascinated by the bodies of the women who seemed not to care or notice the wrinkles and fat that hung from them. In truth, those bodies, so unwieldy and loose, scared me. I wondered why these women didn't hide their bodies like they were expected to. When I would scuttle into the change rooms, dripping from the pool but busting to go to the toilet, I would see them undressing. How could they so proudly show these sorts of bodies in a public space? Did they not understand that they were supposed to be ashamed? That they were disgusting? If I was sure of anything it was that I didn't want to be like this, to not know when I was old and ugly.

Through our giggles and jokes we reinforced a sense of shame about the changes that take place in these bodies. We are made to feel embarrassment about skin that is no longer snug around our muscles. We stop wearing clothing that might expose the sagging and wrinkly body underneath. And we laugh at the women who have no regard for hiding their upper arms.

There is strict policing of women who don't read the signs that their bodies are no longer appropriate for show. 'Mutton dressed as lamb' is how I had heard women described who fail to read the room. They were the women who have an interest in their sexual lives that doesn't match the wrinkles that have begun to gather not only on their faces but now around their knees.

For me, the snood was the beginning of the quiet questioning that happens. Am I just putting on weight? Or is this it? The beginning of the end?

* * *

Maybe our ageing bodies break down ever so slowly so that we might conceive of our end. The decaying provides an opportunity to face the deepest truth of our living: that we will die. The way a healthy body dies, breaking down over years, takes us through a process of release. We can grieve for it slowly throughout the decades as we say goodbye to the experiences or the people our bodies once enabled us to have and be. We can adjust to the new ways we can interact with this world that no longer reflect the image of ourselves we held for so long.

The decaying process is the physical manifestation of our impending erasure. We can see the change that takes place on our skin, feel it in our bones. It's a change that doesn't allow us to hide.

Inside this body, we are in full flight, we are glorious. But this outer form betrays us. It is in freefall from the moment we are born, ageing from that very first breath. The day we arrive on earth we begin to take the journey to our end. We're just somehow tricked into believing it's not like that.

The question we find ourselves inevitably asking about ageing is can we cure or delay it, or make it hard for it to rob us of our precious quality of life? There is endless scientific research about how possible it might be to delay ageing. Is there a way that we can stop this process of decay?

One of three recipients of the 2009 Nobel Prize for physiology was Elizabeth Blackburn, who won the prize for her work understanding telomeres, the little protective tips at the end of chromosomes. Blackburn's work showed that when telomeres wear down over time, they shorten and no longer protect chromosomes, impacting our cellular health. Telomere shortening happens to all of us but at different rates. So can we look after telomeres to ensure they protect our chromosomes for longer? Well, yes, is the short answer. But while the science is prize-winning, the advice is not exactly revelatory: reduce stress, exercise, eat healthy whole foods and get more sleep.

It's the same insights that were gained from the very first large-scale, long-term study done on women in the mid to late years of their lives. The Women's Healthy Ageing Project at the University of Melbourne followed more than four hundred women with the intention of helping women and health professionals understand how to make positive impacts on 'healthy ageing' for women. Cassandra Szoeke, a professor of medicine, doctor, scientist, clinical researcher and expert in women's health, was one of the chief investigators in the study, which commenced in 1990 and focused on women aged forty-five to fifty-five before their transition into menopause. The study accumulated thirty years of data on social connectedness, diet, mood and exercise.

A key takeaway from the study is that exercise and movement are key in living longer and healthier lives, and that the time to start behaviours to aid healthy ageing is in our midlife or before. The study found that it didn't really matter if the exercise was moderate or intense, the main benefit was that the exercise needed to be regular. Maintaining a practice of moving daily assisted the 'cumulative' impact. The study found that as little as fifteen to twenty minutes a day of activity can increase your life span by three to seven years.[1]

The push towards programs that support healthy ageing has received more interest recently as the cost of health has increased due to life spans extending beyond sixty. Economic rationalism saves the day? We understand healthy ageing as a process of developing and maintaining a capacity for wellbeing in older age. To hope to maintain health into older age there is a necessity for people to maintain physical and mental health. But it's essential that the way we understand healthy ageing takes into account the individual's socio-cultural and physical factors.[2]

* * *

Nearly fifty per cent of Australians are living with one or more chronic illnesses. Being ill can make you feel much older than you are and before your time – you're exposed to the world of frailty, of fragility.

Having Crohn's disease for twenty-odd years has lifted the veil for me somewhat on what it means to have a body in decay. For many years I found it hard to get off a chair, roll out of bed or feel like there was any energy at all left in my system – I felt like I had been sucked of everything. And with this change I began to think of myself differently. I needed to quell desires I once might have had for the type of life this body was supposed to provide. It became too tiring to imagine the world of movement; 'quiet and slow' was how I needed to think. While the young girl who lived inside me still wanted to leap and run, she was forced to change the life she had to live.

I know what it feels like when your body starts to break down. When one chronic illness means that you are likely to have another, your morning begins with the ingestion of dozens of tablets in an attempt to find balance for a system that is antagonising itself. It was my introduction to understanding that the inside me and the outside me could be in conflict, and the only resolution to that conflict was a deep and complex process of acceptance.

Throughout my illness there have been long moments of enforced stillness where my body could no longer move without incredible pain. I would lie in a hospital bed and watch people out my window walking through parks or running for the tram. I wanted to go to them to tell them to savour the movement of their bodies, because as with everything, it's often not until something is taken away that we can appreciate aspects of our lives we take for granted.

The disease gave me tiny windows when it would recede from its attack. These momentary lapses in the violence of disease meant that I could find myself back on the track as part of my recovery, running slowly, barely lifting my feet off the ground. It didn't matter anymore how fast this body moved, because at least I was running.

When unwell I would dream about running. I longed for it in a way that surprised me. I remembered that feeling that running gives you – the pain followed by that glorious high. I missed it. I grieved its absence.

Running had such a romantic appeal. I wasn't ever particularly good at it, but I wanted to be. When I started again and every step seemed difficult, I would imagine the running gait of ultramarathon runner Cliff Young, who wore gumboots when he trained on his potato farm in the Otways in Victoria. In 1983, at the age of sixty-one, he won the Sydney to Melbourne Ultramarathon, an 875-kilometre endurance race, and awoke a sleepy, fat Australia into a fevered dream that maybe we could do that too. The image of that man shuffling from Sydney to Melbourne gave us hope that perhaps every crime we had committed against our bodies might be forgiven.

When I started running again, I would pretend I was Cliffy, barely moving my legs and running slowly, just above a walk. It was an attempt to find a kindness again for the body I had cut myself off from. An attempt to feel it again without a fear that the pain would be too much. I had been angry with my body for so long and understood that I needed to find a way to make peace.

Running was a kindness that I was prepared to give it. I would cry with joy at the feeling of aching calf muscles, ecstatic that my body could feel sore because it was moving, not because it was falling apart. Running was a freedom, a body in motion working as it should.

Research supports that it is simple actions that can give our bodies the type of health we long for as we age. There is no silver bullet, but if there were it would be in the form of movement and healthy eating, with fewer sugars and refined carbohydrates. The stuff we've known for decades

The quest to cease the process of ageing has been sought for centuries. To drink from the elixir of youth. To wind back time. To be wise in the body of a young person. These are the dreams that we have been seeking.

We have always been curious to see how far our bodies can take us. How high they can climb. How fast they can run. How long they might fast. Biohacking, or DIYbio, is a term for stuff we've been doing to our bodies forever. It is biological experimentation or 'hacking' that is done by an individual to improve their own biological performance: anything that will mean an individual might be faster, stronger, more relaxed, more focussed or simply more 'alive'. We have always wanted to take the optimisation of our brains and our bodies into our own hands. If we start to lose faith in the power of western medicine or know there is more that we could be doing for ourselves, we might want to seize more control of our biology.

Biohacking is not one single thing or ideology, and therefore encompasses an extensive array of behaviours and experiments. Biohacking can be about fixing illness, being stronger and more mentally efficient, and for some it is about living longer. What might begin with an interest in improving the quality of life becomes a quest for the best quality of life that is possible.

A subgroup of biohackers are the Grinders, who hack their bodies for peak performance by using cybernetic devices. Their aspiration is in becoming cybernetic organisms (aka cyborgs) by utilising gadgets and implants inserted under the skin.[3] Machines being integrated into our bodies is not a new idea. We can think of pacemakers, contraceptive coils and hearing aids as a form of 'transhumanism', a term coined by Julian Huxley (brother of Aldous, author of *Brave New World*) that has come to represent a movement that believes that human beings have a right and an ability to use technology to evolve our species through this augmentation.[4]

It really is the stuff of the future, mixing technology with old wisdoms to heighten the function of biology and slow the process of ageing through ice baths, breathing techniques and electronic implants to name just a few. Biohackers have found fame and fortune by sharing what they claim are successful hacks to reduce some of the more common ailments associated with ageing.

Wim Hof, Dutch-born extreme athlete also referred to as the Ice Man, popularised a breathing technique used by Tibetan monks for centuries called *tummo*. First recorded as part of the six dharmas (the teachings compiled by the Indian mahasiddha Naropa), *tummo*, which translates to 'inner fire', is considered to be the root of the meditation practice. Renamed the Wim Hof method, this popularised breathwork technique has largely extracted the spiritual aspects and visualisations that are central to *tummo*. In doing so, Hof has been able to popularise and make accessible a simple technique that he claims will increase your energy, give you better sleep, reduce your stress levels and encourage a stronger immune system.[5]

But many are not convinced that there is enough done by Wim Hof to temper the hope of some that the technique will be a cure-all. While Wim Hof doesn't advocate that his breathing techniques will cure cancer and other diseases, he does believe it's possible.

Biohacking can range in its intensity and sense of adventure from small changes in the way you live to larger, more invasive changes. The issue the mainstream health industry has with biohacking is that many hacks are unproven or without peer research and validation, which leaves the door open for dangerous outcomes.

But there are many low-risk biohacks, like walking barefoot or the Japanese physiological and psychological exercise of forest bathing – which involves using all of our senses and being present when we spend time in nature. While evidence of the benefits of forest bathing or walking barefoot is still being interrogated, literature reviews are generally positive. Studies that have been undertaken on the physiological effects of shinrin-yoku indicate that forest environments could lower concentrations of cortisol, lower pulse rate, lower blood pressure, increase parasympathetic nerve activity, and lower sympathetic nerve activity.[6] And while there are these interesting physical benefits, it's hard to imagine that encouraging people to walk slowly through the bush can be anything but beneficial.

Swimming in the ocean year-round has become an activity popular with ageing communities around our coasts, where groups of swimmers meet in the early hours of the morning to enjoy the benefits of cold water, community and exercise while anecdotally recording improvements in health. I tried it once when the water was around 10°C and became an instantaneous convert! I felt like I had found the answer I had been looking for. The energy that I received from diving into that water and the exhilaration when I left it were immense. The blood that must have been pumping through me to spark this enormous wave of energy felt incredible.

Biohacking seems to give a sense that we can gain some control in our lives. That we can make decisions about how long we live and are not simply at the mercy of our telomeres or the myriad of biological process that might ultimately go wrong. But it is also a way for us to stave off the anxiety that our mortality brings us, to attempt to avoid an acceptance of the inevitability of our death.

Lisa Leong suffered a debilitating bout of shingles while she was at the top of her game. She was considered successful by those around her. A sprint-distance triathlete and successful commercial lawyer, she had been brought up with the idea that hard work was the formula for success. But once she took a small break, the hard work caught up with her and a bout of shingles rendered her once active body unbearable to the touch. 'I would wince if my child ran towards me, it hurt so much to be touched.'

It was a relentless pain that she had never encountered before. It exposed to her the fragility of her body and the folly that she had believed sheer force would overcome all. 'I just assumed I would just push through everything, but this made me realise that I had a limit. There were red flags but I just ignored them.'

She hunted for ways other people had dealt with such issues. 'I knew I had to do something about my health. I literally couldn't go on the way I was.' Becoming fascinated with the extent that other people were using hacks to improve their health, she submitted to her own experimentation and explored a variety of biohacks that had varying degrees of peer-reviewed scientific evidence. 'Cryotherapy, infrared saunas, hyperbaric oxygen chamber, PEMF mat, acupressure sleep mat, blue blockers, human charger, weirdo glasses that shine green lights into your eyeballs for jet lag ... Some of these I realised were just too intense for my body, and even if there has been scientific research done into them, you'll find that the research hasn't likely been done on a woman.'[7]

Years on, Lisa reports that there are simple hacks she has continued to use and she's the better for it. 'I have a great deal of energy and I reckon I will keep exploring hacks that I run into.' But some things were too intense for her to continue with. 'Some of the hacks I was trying just felt like they were too much for my body.'

While the experience of ageing can be largely cultural, the reality is that what will end us is fundamentally biological. We cannot escape the reality that we are born into a body that will eventually die, even if that death is delayed by extra running sessions, cutting out sugar or integrating technology into our flesh and bones.

We must reckon with this death. Our bodies will age, and they will die.

Air

CHAPTER 7

Stillness: Midlife

THERE IS A PHENOMENON called prairie madness. Anecdotally, it is said to have claimed both the mental health and lives of many early pioneers who set up home on the Great Plains, a broad expanse of flatland in North America. While not an officially documented medical condition, prairie madness was said to be the result of long periods of isolation during which people experienced depression and violent outbursts.

Many historical accounts from the late nineteenth and early twentieth centuries report that the sound of the wind as it screamed mercilessly across this dust bowl was one of the catalysts of this 'madness'. In such isolation and under the stress these early pioneers experienced, listening to the howl of the wind became unbearable.[1,2]

* * *

The most calamitous disasters can happen in total silence. My midlife came upon me like this. It crept up on me in the darkness with such careful steps that I didn't hear it until it had already approached my bed and crawled under the covers. I woke up and had found it had attached itself to me – it had become me. And then the unimaginable loudness when the storm whips up from nowhere, and I am in total darkness.

Be under no illusion – the middle is always the worst place to be. The middle of the back seat in the car when you're a kid, the middle of a fight, the middle of a breakdown. The middle of a meaningless life. The middle section of your ever-expanding body. The middle kid in the family. The middle of the night. The middle of a tornado. And we all know that the middle part of anything sweet is never as good as the end.

It is difficult to know how to prepare to middle out. To have nothing to solve or fix but instead find that you're neck-deep in the confusion of banality. The thickness and sludge of being stuck in a sameness that seems to be on an eternal loop.

I had been taught to be alert for disasters or moments when I might bottom out. I had felt life rush through me in times of disaster when the adrenaline would run just under my skin and make every part of me feel alive. But to middle out? To be lost? No one had taught me how to deal with this wasteland or live in this nothingness space.

It is strange that hitting middle age came as such a shock because I had heard about it since I was a child. I saw it on TV shows, where adults didn't know who they were anymore. Endless movies about parents who were mocked for losing their mojo. We've been told that the searing sense of utter fruitlessness happens to most adults, but we somehow do a brilliant job in avoiding thinking about how it might affect us until it is jammed up against our face.

Like menopause, shrouded in silence, no one really told me how ageing would actually feel, a time when I would need to reckon with where I had found myself.

Everything up until this point had been about striving forward. What did 'not young anymore' women do with this new identity? Was I now allowed to talk about myself as an older woman? Was that disrespectful to women who were older than me? Could I discuss how it felt like a smarting slap across the face or would this corner me, make me seem vain and without the fortitude of feminists determined that we should be proud of these ageing selves?

When it hits, it can be consuming. Finally, it seems, we have come to properly understand the machinations of the world and realise that nothing really matters. We begin to see the game for what it is: one that we were never meant to win but one where the winning is not the purpose. But in this confused state, how do we avoid impulsive decisions that we hope might bring life back into the depths of the apathy that claw at every cell, that might only work to blow everything up?

This loss is disorienting, like loss often is. No warning. No time to prepare. Just suddenly your young self is gone, lifted up by the wind and relocated. No trace. No funeral. Just disappeared, sudden enough to warrant your face being plastered on the back of milk cartons: *Missing – have you seen her?*

We are matter moving through space and time. Ageing happens to us both as a reality of biology and a construct of culture. We move slower, our skin sags and our organs get tired. We harbour disease and illness like an armed shipwreck on the bottom of an ocean ready to detonate with the slightest movement. But mostly we are coerced, convinced even, into how to see ourselves as we age. We are told how we fit or don't fit into the broad and powerful whole. We are seen in a contrast-and-compare kind of way, relative to another. Age, I am starting to understand, is always relative, and there are always younger people whom we are thrust up against and told, 'See? Different.'

I would look back over old photos and compare them with how I looked now. 'Would you notice that I had changed?' I wondered. How old would you think I was? And I would go out of my way to hear someone tell me that they thought I looked young for my age. 'Yes!' I would silently proclaim. 'I'm not old now ... perhaps I never will be,' I quietly hoped.

We had a sense of the fruitlessness of life when we were teenagers. When we were young we knew we had to agitate on the edges. Never conform, we promised. Keep pushing back at the absurdity of the world that we had been born into. None of it made sense back then, but it seems they get to most of us eventually. We're sucked into the mundanity of the everyday. We end up playing the game so that we won't get left behind.

I think I knew I had hit the middle when I stopped wondering about the world around me. There was a boredom and a belief that I had already seen it all. I forgot to look, to really see what was before me. Hitting the middle was met with a feeling of losing that buzz you get when you see something for the first time, the many exhilarating moments of firsts. Of discovery. Of finding out how your skin feels against the world. Of what it means to live in your body. Of love and loss and the exhilaration of dancing through the night.

When you find yourself suddenly in the middle, you've got to work out how to read the tea leaves that tell when and how it actually happened. To begin with, there is a lot of speculation. They think I'm old. Is that what's going on? Should I be wearing this now? Can I want for things the way I used to? Do they think I shouldn't be here? Can I want to look younger than I am?

It is a seismic shift in the way you are now allowed to see and understand yourself. One of the things we have always been aware of when we see people age around us is that a lack of awareness of your age relative to others is embarrassing. More horrific than ageing is if you don't realise that you are. You worry the kids will laugh behind your back or roll their eyes at your total misunderstanding of how the world now is, so you're alert to any movement in the bushes. Do they think I'm old?

Recently I was at a bar and started a great conversation with a stranger. It wasn't long before we were holding each other's arms as we ferociously agreed about the terms of living. Then midway through the conversation she said words that are still reverberating through me today: 'I wish you could adopt me and be my mum.' I stepped back slightly and covered my shock with a laugh and an enthusiastic nod. 'Of course, I'd love to be your mum,' I said.

Her bloody mum? How old did I look to her? Did she think I was capable of giving birth when I was ... well, I guess the maths sort of worked out. I looked in the mirror and tried to see myself as someone else might. To my eye I was still that young girl who looked back at herself when she was five ... and fifteen and thirty-five. But now, well beyond those years, was I ageing? That mythical experience we have heard whispered in dark corridors. It's other people that it happens to. Other people we've seen with walking sticks and wrinkles since we were children.[3]

* * *

I had always been taught that life was a straight line. Of course it's not, or at least it shouldn't be, but there is a great pressure to conform to a life as if it can be done in some sort of recognisable sequence. You're told to go to school, then get a job, maybe travel if you can afford to, partner up and have a child and then, somewhere further down that line, you die. And on this fictional straight path, part of the ageing process is coming to terms with the fact that while you are still heading forward, without much warning there will be a middle point when the journey flips and you find that you are now heading towards the end.

There must be a middle point you cross that changes the meaning of your journey. And it was realising that I'd crossed that point, probably years before, and had been travelling not as someone who had left the beginning, but as someone who was heading towards the end, that I found devastating.

This middle point can be fertile ground for a crisis when we realise that we are hurtling towards our end. I could smell it in the air, a rancid odour telling me that nothing I had poured my energy into had really been worth it. That all the time I had spent building a life, waiting for its ultimate triumph to emerge, had likely already passed its golden moment. The rest was going to be downhill.

Worse are the times when it is seen by others before you, when someone points out that you are old before you know it to be who you are. When you are regarded as old because someone has stood up for you on the train. Or kids explain something as though you couldn't possibly understand the technical detail – and then simultaneously you realise that, yes, in fact you could not possibly understand the technical detail.

I was once doing a music interview with someone I didn't consider much younger than me. I certainly didn't expect that he would perceive me to be much older than him. During the interview he started to talk about the relevance of Pokémon in his music, and I was nodding along as if this was something I spoke to my friends about on the regular. He stopped halfway through and clarified that Pokémon was something that had been important to his generation – did I know what they were?

My eyebrows shot up in a defensive retort. 'Of course I do,' I spat. But in truth I had no idea. I didn't really understand what he was talking about, not really. I had seen them but understood nothing of their relevance to culture. I was horrified that he would see me as an outsider to his life. Weren't we the same? 'Shit. You reckon I'm old.'

* * *

There is a myriad of articles written about the midlife crisis. Lists on how to avoid it. One of the most wonderful suggestions I read in one such survival guide was simply 'Don't have an affair'.[4] And perhaps it is a simple as that – don't do it. But when I caught up with Anjali, a woman who had recently been grappling with what she felt had been a midlife crisis, it is, of course, not that simple.

I met Anjali for the first time at a bar on a weeknight after I had found her story online. We looked like a lot of other middle-aged women that night, and most other nights of the week. We were huddled close and discussing where we felt it had gone wrong. She began giving me some of the earlier details of her life – her parents had been migrants, were in love and had stayed married until her mum died three years ago. She had met her partner at university and she had been happy with him for most of their relationship. It had been easy, and he had been there for her during a recent health scare.

But things had started to change. The easiness of their relationship had started to feel less easy and more like it had become boring. There was nothing left to surprise each other, they had been down every road imaginable together. She had assumed that her mothering and her job as a lawyer had covered her almost entirely. She felt suffocated and alone.

'I realised that I was living deep in my imagination,' she said. 'It must have been a midlife crisis. I was somewhere else in my imagination. I was imagining that I was someone else, I guess. Or maybe I was imagining who I used to be.'

It happens often when we want to believe we have a handle on our lives. When we are unconscious or in denial of the existential pain we must be in. So when someone offers us some relief, it doesn't even feel as if it is a choice – it feels as if it might be the only way we might find ourselves again.

Her relief came in the form of a younger man she had started working with. 'He sought me out,' she said. 'I can't tell you now even why, but he definitely made a beeline for me, and we became close friends really quickly.' We order another beer. 'It got to the point where I loved sharing my time with him – because I guess suddenly I felt seen. I felt with him like I used to feel. I had no interest in a relationship with him, it wasn't like that, and he didn't want one with me. It was just having that level of friendship that I had missed, I think. It woke me up to what I had been grieving.'[5]

There are endless lists of red flags provided in those glossy magazines to let you know when you've entered midlife: apathy, sleeplessness, boredom. But one that really resonated with me was 'an overwhelming sense of loss'.[6] I had first noticed this years ago. I felt it creep up inside me and then one day it felt fully formed. It was almost an impossible grief, a painful tug that sat in my chest and told me that at almost every conceivable level, every possible way I could approach it, the world was painful. Love was painful. Loss was painful. Living in between loss and love was painful. It barely seemed possible to survive the feeling of such deep grief. I felt like my illness had robbed years of my life. Had I missed out on being who I might have been because of years in hospitals and a life spent laying sick in bed? The irreversibility of this time. The realisation that I wasn't going to get it back really hurt.

The midlife is a crisis because we are so utterly unprepared for it. And while there are endless lists to tell you how to avoid a midlife crisis, there are also endless lists for if you've found yourself neck-deep in a midlife crisis and how you might climb your way out. There are self-help pieces that tell you how to reinvigorate your life without blowing it into smithereens. The temptation, of course, is to change everything – your partner, your job, your body – in the hope that you might breathe life back into what once felt alive.

How do these changes happen in us? How can we be swept away from where we have been moored? When we suddenly find ourselves in the middle of a rip, with no knowledge of how to get back to shore, questioning everything that has led us there?

Is there a metric to realise you're in your midlife? Is it an age? Or do we wait to be told? Midlife could really be anywhere from thirty-five years of age onwards. The midpoint of a career. Or of a life spent parenting. Or of the myriad of things we do to explain to people what we believe we 'are'.

Perhaps midlife could be described as the time when seeking and discovery has hit a natural point where it must find a way to continue to propel forward, or we will sink down and be lost. But suddenly it all seems so pointless. What was this all about? you wonder.

What felt like an eternal journey to find yourself in the world suddenly hits a point where you have perhaps arrived, and it doesn't feel quite as you'd hoped. This was the time when I was faced with not only the idea of my physical death but the death of my identity as relevant in this new world that had built up around me.

No one seems excited about the people who live in the middle. We're not feisty octogenarians wearing brightly coloured glasses and outrageous clothes telling everyone our secret is sipping whisky under a full moon. And we're certainly not the beautiful young people whose skin shines. We are the frumpy middle, like a large expanse of road that sits between towns – just something to be endured until we finally arrive somewhere else.

* * *

The midlife understood as being a crisis was invented in 1957 on a nondescript day in London by Canadian psychoanalyst Dr Elliott Jaques. When he presented his paper to a bunch of other mind doctors, he was talking about a midlife that would happen to someone in their thirties. Eight years later, when he published another paper called 'Death and the mid-life crisis', the world was ready and raring to adopt the idea of an existential crisis that one faces when realising that death happens to them, not that old person who lives down the road.[7]

These days your thirties seem a little early for a midlife crisis, but a recent Household, Income and Labour Dynamics in Australia (HILDA) survey confirms that life starts to feel a little less satisfying when we hit our thirties and we're probably at our most dissatisfied as we make our way through our forties and fifties. Many researchers and philosophers have grappled with why. Why is life so unsatisfying at this midpoint? Perhaps it is about that endless amount of hope that sits somewhere inside you when you're young, and when every drop of that hope has been used up, there doesn't feel like there is much point anymore. You've done everything you set out to do, and if you didn't, it's too late, we think.[8]

To think back and realise that I had once believed there was an actual destination suddenly seemed foolish. Instead, I was finding out that there was just an endless sameness of sand in every direction. There were no longer landmarks that I could anchor to, and I was rushed with the panic that comes when you realise you might very well be lost. Lost like in the dreams I would have regularly when a crushing nothingness would take my breath away, a darkness so deep and impenetrable that I ceased to be.

Who are you in this landscape? Everything you have known of yourself and how you relate to the world has been transformed somehow, the tricks we play to allow the ego to feel relief no longer at our disposal. Our hair is falling out, our faces are looking worn, we no longer have the energy we once did, and the world makes sure we know it. Barely an eyebrow is lifted when we enter the room. We are mediocrity personified.

It had all felt so clear moments ago. I guess I had been convinced to at least try to travel on that straight line. So many years with your head down, working hard, maybe bringing up a couple of kids, paying off debts, relying on the unreliability of the world, partnering, divorcing, breaking, fixing and finding out that it never stops. Realising there isn't a moment when you get a knock on the door and are informed that you've made it.

When I realised that I was lost somewhere in the middle I was filled with panic and apathy. I had simultaneous urgent desires to both run and sleep. I wanted to change. To be more. To be less. To be the same as I used to be. To be entirely new. To go back somehow. To reverse some of the decisions. Why had I been so afraid?

This whole idea of reaching the summit is really just about coming back down the long and steep descent. There is a massive party for you at the top. *Congratulations* is the sign they've stuck on a post. *Well done!* But you understand that this is a party for an end, not a beginning. You have come as far as you're ever going to. The rest is now a journey to a finish line. And heading down is going to be much faster than the effort it took to get there in the first place.

Oldness is repulsive, we're taught. We come to understand the ageing form as the end of something. Oldness is about the end of life, where we lie down and endure for the decades when we eventually are understood as old.

To discard us, to make the job as palatable as possible, we have all been taught to despise our form, so we can perform the exorcism without guilt. That is why we have cast old women as witches and intolerant old biddies who are utterly sexless and who try to steal the youth and beauty of other women.

* * *

This feeling was finally described during Covid-19 and lockdowns as a sense of languishing, where you feel a little lost at sea. Days roll together and become indistinguishable from the one before. We languish because we can lose that connection, that deep hum inside us, guiding us towards something that has real meaning.

What had all this rushing about to get somewhere been about? And where had I been heading anyway? No one saw me as someone who might be emerging in the world. My friend Kirsty looked at me with her big, questioning eyes that I have always loved, 'I'm honestly so scared. I'm over fifty, no one wants women who are over fifty. What's going to happen if I can't get a job? What am I going to do? Go back to school?'

The spirit that drove us to keep getting up when we got knocked down, that eternal feeling of hope, is tired. It has lost its momentum, its purpose, its meaning. It is the electricity of birth that we miss. The birth of new ideas. New ways to explore our humanity. New smells. New foods. New things to touch. The blood that drips off our lips because we bit down too hard. I even missed the failures. The devastations.

Instead, it felt like it had all been explored. Every first I was ever going to have had been done. Now I felt that I was in the depths of winter, where the winds were howling outside so that I couldn't leave, and I was looking at a long stretch of time stuck inside, wondering how the hell I had arrived here. And am I ever getting out?

But I had read how important it is to appreciate the winters of our lives. The literal winters and the metaphoric ones. To lie down and rest. There is nothing to be done outside; it is too cold. It is time to repair. Winter is a time when we slow down so we can gather ourselves. To reflect on the world outside our door and to ready ourselves for the warmer weather to come.

Whether we like it or not, the winter and the wild winds outside our door will demand our respect. I knew there would be no avoiding this lesson. Those who had tried to resist this time had found this a crisis as they lurched from disaster to disaster. Midlife ensured I would respect that this was the time for a serious moment of stillness. Of quiet. Of facing the demons of all the artifice that I had spent so much time building up around me, because I thought it might keep me safe. Ideas of myself that were not capable of persisting through this next part of my life. I had to sleep it off and hope to wake to something that was different.

This was the first battle and I knew there was no option but surrender. I understood that ageing and this moment of midlife would only be about renewal if I was prepared to lose it all so that I might find myself again. That the moments of firsts might return if I was prepared to see myself reflected back as something new. To see myself again for the first time. It was time for me to lie down, cover myself in the dirt and the mud, while the wind screamed outside my door. And breathe in deeply. In and out. In. Out. And close my eyes. What might I be when I wake up? I wondered, while my heart beat with hope for what might emerge.

Air

CHAPTER 8

Sirocco: Mirror, Mirror

I REALISED IT WAS probably me who was perpetuating these 'old' ideas of myself. Midlife easily takes a foothold in our consciousness and self-perception because we have been warming up to these concepts of age for a long time. In fact, I realised I was likely the one who had done most of the work to make sure that I felt lost when I became 'old'.

'You're fat, look at you …' I heard whispered from what seemed like somewhere far away. 'Look at those wrinkles. You're old.' It continued uninterrupted, and I realised it wasn't coming from outside, it was there inside me, where my breath smells black. 'You're an ugly thing, you are.'

I had heard these incantations so many times when I looked in the mirror that I didn't notice them much anymore. Not really. It wasn't like I listened to them anyway. The words had transformed into a dull thrum that had found a home deep inside me, where the black flowers grew. If you asked me to find them, I couldn't. They had leaked into me and were now just a song on loop, flowing like a river through every part of me.

Incantations like these don't need a language. They might start that way, songs we've heard sung to us by the magpies that we repeat in whispers as we drift off to sleep. But they take a form inside us and become part of our bodies, our blood. They beat inside our hearts like an incubus that convinces its host that it belongs.

I leant in as close to my reflection as I could bear and focused hard to keep my gaze steady. The light in the bathroom was soft, making this job at least possible. I was irritated to look again, but this was rote, nearly as familiar as breathing.

Spots, red patches, bags, wrinkles, stray hairs, uneven tones, misshapen, discoloured. I can see the fat that has gathered around my chin so that now there are two of them. Sometimes when I have looked I think I see a teenage boy. I have often tiptoed out to someone else to double-check – did they see it too? Did I look like a boy to them?

When I was young I would look longingly at the skater boys I knew. They were always boys when I was growing up. Baggy pants rolled up with flat sneakers. An oversized t-shirt and dirty hair. I longed to look like them. To be so unaware of any responsibility to my form. To be innocent of that kind of corruption. I have begun to edge my way there sometimes, the utter freedom of disappearing inside some clothing. Invisible.

'Who are you?' I would often wonder. It didn't look like me in the mirror, or at least I didn't really want the me I thought I knew to look like this. The person who lives inside this body doesn't know what she looks like until she sees her reflection. If you asked me to, I couldn't recall my image, not really. I could give you basic details – hair, eye colour – but that's about it. Not even if I close my eyes and think about the millions of times that I have seen her, I simply can't picture her – well, not the way she ends up looking here, anyway, in the mirror.

It had always been curious to me how the outside didn't match the inside. How old did I feel deep inside my bones? Did I feel like the me who was young and alive twenty, thirty, forty years ago? Or was I this older woman who was staring back? I couldn't tell.

Often I don't feel like a girl at all; instead I feel neutral and wild and without boundaries. I feel full with the possibilities that disturb the butterflies that live in my stomach, because I still harbour hope that there is more for me somehow. When I stare deep into my eyes, I don't really recognise who is looking back at me. I don't know what I imagine I am, but it's not this.

I breathe in hard. I am tired of being looked at and I'm tired of looking. Every single day, multiple times a day, for decades, I have been looking. Looking but not really seeing. What would happen if I stopped? If one day, I just stopped looking. If I got out of bed, got dressed and brushed my hair, all without regarding the girl that lives inside the mirror. She's hostile and, quite frankly, a bad start to my day – why should I be paying her so much attention?

So as soon as I have finished looking, I try to forget how it felt. To erase the disappointment. To go back to the image of me that I have constructed somewhere else, the image that includes how it *feels* to be me, full of colour and movement. Of fight and resistance. And I continue with the day as if none of those concerns are mine, because of course I am beyond that sort of vanity. I try to meld with a sense of me that doesn't have a knowledge of how this body looks.

The objectification that had been a central point of my life for such a long time was a significant aspect in trying to understand this transition. Objects – good objects, at least – have some sort of utility. Even if the point of an object is to be aesthetically pleasing, it remains valuable. After the body has been used for its purpose, the body, the object, no longer serves a need.

If you've never been an object, it may be difficult to understand how subject and object can merge. How the insistence that you are an object has a certain pervasive power over you. That somehow you begin to believe you are exactly what they've said you are. You embody the way you are seen.

When the subject also performs the objectification, we are lost somewhere in between. The darkness between subject and object is where we are forced to reside, where we are truly neither. We live in the world in between, hoping that one day we might emerge and be found again as young as the day we went into hiding. Like a perfectly preserved fossil.

* * *

We have always longed to see our reflection. To know what this body that we live inside truly looks like. To see how it fits in with all the bodies that live around us. To be simultaneously subject and object, seen and the seer – to be the judge and the judged.

At first we had to make do with reflections found in our natural world. And then later, seeing yourself was only for those with rank or wealth. There was status in having your image reproduced, staid impressions of the human form captured standing utterly still, the life breathed out of them.[1]

When I take a photo, I find myself holding my breath so that the animation in my body is stilled and the camera can capture a moment that only seems like it is me. The smile. The tilt of the head. We practise how it looks when we do it. Then we check back on the digital camera and see if we like what we have created. If not, we ask to do it again, this time shifting slightly to the left and tilting to avoid the ugly.

I am so closely aligned with the sharp image that is staring back at me – so deeply do I think I am what I see – that I believe those flaws and failings have been born into me. They have buried themselves into my fabric and become the black breath that exhales from me. The flaws that I perceive on the outside I believe to be the flaws of my very deepest self.

Until a discovery by German chemist Justus von Liebig as recently as 1835 made the modern mirror widely available, we hadn't seen ourselves with the sharp focus that we do now. Ancient Egyptians, the Mayans and the ancient Chinese used highly polished copper, obsidian or lead, but these mirrors were only capable of reflecting twenty per cent of the available light. What did they make of themselves as they were straining through the murkiness to see their human form?[2]

These days the image is so clear that as we lean in we can see the tiny hairs on our skin. The divots and pores. The black spots of imperfection. The sharpened image feels like you might be able to look back through time to the self that set eyes upon itself when you were a child, just as Dorian Gray did, who took the opportunity to give up his soul so that he might be granted eternal youth.[3]

Why is the bargain for youth always done with the devil? Faust is the earliest and most enduring depiction of a man's desperate bargain to remain young. We sense that our desire for youth is morally questionable. We sense that our hunger is that of the ego. And we are ashamed of it. But we would give away everything for eternal youth.[4]

As soon as I had seen her in this mirror, I was afraid not to look. Would she be more disgusting if I didn't check on her and brush and clean her? Would she be overrun by the thoughts and impressions that others have of her? If I didn't see her each and every day, what might happen to her? Would she be lost?

The moment we gaze upon our image we become complicit with the outside world and its agenda. We become an agent of its falsity and, perhaps unwittingly, we agree to the terms that the self is loved or lost in that reflection. We engage in the ritual of the observer and the observed. We become our own keepers, ready to scrutinise our own image before anyone else does. We dig and pull and push the person in that reflection, hunting for all the ways that we might not be loved. We seek to find any hint of failure so that we can eradicate it. Or be buried by it.

I guess I believed that if I attacked myself first, I might avoid the pain of a surprise attack from outside. And I would wonder if I could try to hide what was happening to me. To colour. To shine. To peel. To cut and rearrange. When I looked at myself in the mirror, that's what I was mostly looking for – the ways I could avoid being lost forever in that reflection.

But I realised I couldn't avoid her. My reflection shows up everywhere. Even when I least expect it, she is there. I see her when I drive, when I walk past windows, I see her in phones and on my social media feed. I see her reflected back in nature. I am constantly in receipt of myself. I am severed into both the person who is watching and the person who is being watched.

It wasn't always this way. There was a glorious time when we were simply unaware that we lived inside us. When is it that we realise the person in the mirror is the same person who lives inside our skin? Research suggests that the process of knowing ourselves as bodies begins as early as seven months and that we can recognise ourselves as the 'me' in a mirror at around eighteen months.[5]

I have always wondered who I was before I could see the reflection of myself and know it as me. Did I know myself just by the way I *felt*? Before I first saw myself and knew it as 'me', how was I created in my mind? Was I simply a memory of that feeling when I first felt the dirt rub against my feet? The wetness of the earth, the coldness hard up against my soles? Was I the air that ran across my legs, that caused my skin to goosebump? Or the sunlight that burnt slightly on my cheeks, warming my skin? Or my own fingernails that cut against me?

Was I the ocean that rose and fell inside me? The rush and crash of excitement and terror that coursed through my veins? Or was I the smell of the lavender bush that took me back instantly to the time when my mum forgot to pick me up from school? Or the sound of the bell that rang inside me, bouncing off my bones, absorbing into my flesh, telling me it was time to go inside?

There is a moment when that reflection and the self become fused, and somehow the inside and the outside feel as if they are same thing. Before then, when we don't conceive that there is a separate self at all, it is a matter of *learning* our bodies. As babies, we map our bodies piece by piece, so that each part of our body corresponds with a certain part of our brain.[6] And when we learn our bodies, we begin to learn the bodies of others. My feet – your feet. My cheeks – your cheeks. It is through our bodies that we learn we are human together, that we are the same. And as I reach out and long for you, this is how it feels when my lips touch your lips. And when your hand touches my hair. We know each other through the way our energy feels inside our bodies when they rub against each other. We know a caress like we know how it feels to be hit.

When we are babies, we hunger for touch as much as we hunger for food. Touch is the way we come to know and understand that we have a body that exists in the world. Touch is the way we learn to speak of love. Our first moment of communication is when our skin feels the skin of another. Our first language is touch.

Before we know ourselves to be that person in the mirror, we hold our hands up to the light and wonder why we feel as we do. We put one chubby finger between our lips as the saliva drips over our knuckles and down our hands. We learn we are hard things that knock up against the world. We are inside something, and somehow that something is us.

Before we have learnt our bodies, we know ourselves as flowing through every part of the world. In fact, there is no world outside because the world as we know it lives inside us. We don't begin or end inside our skin. We are limitless. The body outside is merely a transport vehicle. Don't believe you are the car. You're just in the car.

A study published in 2018 by the University of Washington Institute for Learning and Brain Sciences showed it was possible to measure the specific networks of a baby's brain where the body is represented. The study also showed how babies' brains respond to seeing another person being touched in the absence of being touched themselves. Researchers discovered that even if the baby is simply observing another person being touched, the baby's own somatosensory cortex (the 'touch centre' in the baby brain) also became activated.[7]

We learn about ourselves not only in our own reflection but through how we are reflected by those around us. We are given a sense of who we are by how others see us and make assumptions about us, their ideas mediated solely through our bodies. And so it does matter that they can see *all* of us. It does matter that they can see through our skin and travel deep with us towards the person who lives inside. It does matter if they are limited and can only see what is shown to them on the outside of us.

Even more puzzling is whether I see what you're seeing when you look at me. Are we ever really perceiving ourselves as we are seen? How can we see with the eyes of someone who loves us, who knows the self that resides inside us? Surely they employ something different from the nasty critical disdain we often use to view ourselves.

I unexpectedly walked past a mirror in a shop the other day, and for a few glorious seconds I didn't recognise the me looking back. I saw myself as one might if they weren't embedded in the experience of looking and being looked at. For just a moment I was the object but not the subject. Any hopes that I may have brought to the mirror for it to reflect me in certain ways were absent. I saw myself as I might see anyone through my eyes. And I was just a woman, standing in a shop, shocked that someone was looking straight back at her.

* * *

For the first time in my life I had tried to really look at myself in the mirror. To see myself without the baggage that I would carry to it. To be honest and kind to whoever it was that was looking back at me.

I had read somewhere that every time you are in front of a mirror, you should look into your eyes and say, 'I love you.' The first time I tried, I whispered it, hoping that no one would hear me uttering this weird meditation. As soon as the words came out, I was filled with a strange disgust. An embarrassment at such cheesy sentiments.

I had previously spent my mirror routine creating distractions and daydreams. Hurried glances that only took in some of my reflection. Not enough of me for the full weight of the truth about the state of my skin or the lack of lustre of my hair, but just enough to ensure I'd rubbed in my foundation.

At some point during my teenage years I had developed a 'mirror face'. So deeply practised is it that even though I have tried, I can't stop my face contorting whenever I see a mirror. I haven't seen my real face for decades, not without it being stretched and sucked. As soon as I see my reflection anywhere, I instinctively suck in my nose.

I was eight years old and lining up for the sixty-metre hurdles. I can remember the big gumtrees that surrounded the athletics track I raced at every Saturday morning and the feeling of electricity in my body as I pushed myself against the world to run as fast as I could. I loved the drama, the feeling that it was me against everyone, and all I had were my little legs and arms to pump myself faster. Faster.

Standing beside me was a girl I thought was sweet. I liked the way she smelt and her hair bounced when she ran. As we lined up, about to jump the hurdles, she turned to me, and I was excited to be noticed. 'Do many people tease you about your nose?' she asked, eyebrows high and a genuine sadness in her eyes. And I do believe, in that moment, she did actually feel pain and regret for me and my nose. 'Oh,' I said, laughing. 'Not that much.' I turned away so she couldn't see that I was about to cry. What was she talking about? No one had even mentioned my nose to me before. But from that day, that's the nose I saw in the mirror. The nose she told me I had. A nose that she assumed people would laugh at.

Also interesting is that the hyper-personal impact of being objectified as it plays out in front of my mirror might not even be as a result of personal objectification. Barbara Fredrickson and Tomi-Ann Roberts, psychologists and academics, developed 'objectification theory' in the mid-1990s to understand how women are affected by cultures that objectify the body.[8] The theory defines the process of self-objectification, whereby individuals assume an observer's perspective of their body and place undue emphasis on their appearance. In further research, Tomi-Ann Roberts found that self-objectification stems from sexual objectification and that it leads to negative emotional responses for women, including anxiety and shame.[9]

Technology has ensured that we are now the masters of our own objectification. Selfie culture has been exhaustingly analysed, mainly as a mechanism to deride the play and interrogation of the form of the teenager, by the teenager. But their freedom as the directors of their imagery has been a significant development in the impact of self-objectification. No longer are we in the hands of the voyeur asking us to shift and place our hands in certain ways, to be seen in certain light, to be more pleasingly photographed in certain angles. Now we design these parameters ourselves. The image of the teenage girl soon became a ubiquitous one – she would hold the camera high, turn her cheek slightly to one side and pucker her lips. Soon every photo of a teenage girl looked like this.[10]

* * *

I had read about a woman who had stopped looking into mirrors in the lead-up to her wedding day, inspired by an order of nuns in Renaissance Italy with strict restrictions against vanity. She was aware of the severe criticism that she was whispering to herself when she looked at her reflection; 'too fat and too ugly' was how it sounded in her head. For an entire year she avoided looking. No one thought that this was a good idea, the assessment was that she would struggle without seeing herself, especially for her wedding. But her experience was the opposite. When she finally finished the experiment and looked at her image again, she was happy with what she saw.[11]

In an era when we have moved a lot of our work online, it's actually very hard to find a straight seven days when you are not looking at yourself in one way or another. Women have reported to me feeling less confident than they had in a long time now that they were required to attend online meetings for large parts of their day. Constantly viewing themselves and being aware that others were also viewing them made for some serious self-critique. What would it feel like if we had no idea how we looked? To surrender to the world without having control over what other people were looking at?

After some fruitless digging to find a case study that might be good to speak to this idea, it occurred to me that maybe I should be giving it a go myself. So I made a pledge: no mirrors, no photos, no online meetings where I could see my image. I would avoid objectifying myself for seven days.

The idea made me giddy. I had never known myself without a reference point that existed outside me.

When I started, I had to constantly remind myself to look away if there was a mirror in view. I needed to be ready, because there were mirrors everywhere, in the bathroom, the bedroom, even one as a splashback in our kitchen. The lift in my apartment has one. The entranceway to my building has one. My car has several. I walk past reflections in windows from my car to work. There are mirrors in the bathrooms at work.

I sensed that this was going to be liberating. I decided to do my normal routine but without looking at myself and judging. On the first morning, leaving the bathroom after moisturising, I walked up to my husband. 'Is it all rubbed in?' He looked vaguely up at my face. 'It looks good,' he said, no doubt sensing any other answer would likely get him an unwanted reaction. We'd been here many times before. 'Are you sure?' I asked sceptically. He looked again, this time with more interest. 'Yep, top notch.'

He had been looking at this face for a couple of decades now; I'm not sure even what he sees when he looks at me. I don't think my face is what he has stuck around for and likely not what got him interested in the first place. And while that might sound obvious, it was a significant first thought on this. Perhaps I was more than my face.

The entire day, I dodged my reflection – I was ready to join the resistance. The week felt remarkably like that first day. I felt everything I had hoped to feel. And I didn't miss looking at myself. I especially didn't feel like I had lost my power in the world. In fact, it was the opposite. Just like my husband, it seemed that my face, how I looked, wasn't seen by those outside me as I thought it was. No one really cared in the way I thought they did. It was me who had been imbuing it with the meaning that I believed it had. I was wrong. No one saw me in any way that I might understand.

It was clear that my brand of self-objectification has harmed me more than any objectification I may have received in the world outside. Of course, they are linked, and they flow between each other. Women who have been disregarded or ridiculed in the world will in turn disregard and ridicule themselves. But getting older, perhaps, is about the opportunity to right that wrong. To change the way in which we see ourselves.

The truth is, I don't know what is being seen, but having myself absent from the judgement each morning meant that the voice demanding attention wasn't there to start my day.

The invisibility that we experience as older women could be that first gateway to true emancipation. The fact that no one cares about you anymore enables a certain kind of freedom. And just like the bride who had stopped looking at her reflection for an entire year, when I looked at myself in the mirror at the end of my experiment, it was like I was seeing an old friend. I had a warmth and genuine love for that little face looking back. The absence of my critical objectification for even a short amount of time made me feel different.

* * *

But this voyeurism and self-objectification can also be a source of empowerment, an opportunity to break with the paradigm of beauty and project images that have not been allowed a place in the public domain. Our highly curated worlds have been shaken up by the emergence of imagery that has defied the cultural elite's curation. Now that we can propagate ideas of ourselves and are no longer being policed by the editors of high-end fashion magazines and their commercial interests, there has been an emergence of images that speak of us in a different way.

Melissa Blake blew up the internet in 2019 when she posted three selfies. Difficult to imagine how that is possible – unless, of course, you are a disabled woman and your image, by virtue of your disability, is unavoidably political. As a writer, Melissa Blake had recently published an op-ed on Donald Trump that unleashed a barrage of troll activity on her social media accounts.

Many comments were along these lines: 'you should be banned from posting a picture of yourself because you're too ugly'. Having been on the receiving end of this sort of trolling for a long time, Melissa Blake decided that she was done with taking this lying down. So she launched #mybestselfie and posted a selfie every day for a year.

Her self-crafted images tell a different, unseen story about beauty and of objectification. 'Sometimes I wonder if I should stop posting so many selfies. But then I'm reminded of our reality in 2020: Disabled people have to fight to be seen and heard. These selfies are for every single disabled person who continues to fight every single day.'[12]

I realised that her selfies challenged my own long-held ideas of beauty and, more importantly, a belief that had made its way deep inside me that we have no right to perform a pride in ourselves if we don't fit into the narrow definitions that beauty standards project.

When Melissa Blake posted selfies and declared herself to be 'cute', it gave all of us an opportunity to feel our own pride.

It made us question our own internalised ableism and sexism. We had been silenced, along with her. If we weren't 'told' we were beautiful, we had no right to declare it.[13]

'I may have started this year of selfies for myself,' she wrote, 'but I soon realised that these selfies weren't just about me. Other disabled people told me they identified with my words, too, and they began posting selfies of their own. They started sharing their stories and showing the world who they were. I've often felt very alone as a disabled person and for the first time, I was seeing the disability community taking our rightful place at society's table. Finally, I was seeing people like me – people who weren't ashamed of who they are – and it was one of the most glorious things I've ever experienced.'[14]

More recently, Melissa Blake received a message from a troll who shared with her a screenshot of an internet search. She responded, '[W]ow, troll … you just had to let me know that my photo is one of the first to come up when you Google "ugly fat woman." Sigh, I may play it cool, but I still have insecurities and how I look is something I've always been self-conscious about. I wish I wasn't, but I am …'[15]

The abusive tweet makes it clear that no matter how many moves are made to advance a different narrative about our worth, there is a powerful campaign to ensure we are never too far away from being put back in our place. Melissa Blake, who has done so much to advocate for the experience of disabled women so that we might feel pride, is hunted and attacked. She is mocked and ridiculed. The stronger we seem, the more violent the attacks will be against us. They want us to believe that we can never win. And maybe they're right.

Air

CHAPTER 9

Beaufort: The Scale

INVENTED BY AN IRISH hydrographer named Francis Beaufort, the Beaufort scale measures wind intensity. It's not entirely scientific, but more observational, initially not detailing the wind speeds but the subjective experience of the wind and its impact on the ocean or land.

But it does a good job of understanding that the world is interconnected and that we're not just a set of separate metrics that can ignore the impact on the environment in which we are housed. It begins with a description of the wind as: 'Calm – Sea like a mirror. Calm; smoke rises vertically' and explores the stages of intensity until it arrives at 'Hurricane: Devastation.'[1]

* * *

I have benefited so much from the disability community and advocates like Melissa Blake who expose and push back against the impacts of ableism and a discrimination that is internalised and fosters shame and self-limiting ideas. When we don't match the way we've been told we should look, sound or be in the world, we dutifully restrict ourselves. Through a myriad of images proliferated in media and advertising reinforcing what is acceptable, we internalise shame when we do not match what we see. We have been taught to only love ourselves as far as we relate to the image we've been told is 'normal'.

When I had an ileostomy bag, I felt ugly, as though I had been disfigured and that I would be frightening to anyone who might get too close. There were no images affirming my body and the way my appearance had been transformed by medication. I had internalised ableist ideas of *beautiful* and it took me a long time to find a way back to a love of me. There is such a strong relationship between beauty and worth that I had internalised a shame of who I thought I was.

Beauty columnist Funmi Fetto remembers visiting makeup counters with her Caucasian friends growing up. 'I moved towards the foundations and chose the darkest shade. It was called "Biscuit". I looked like I had white chalk on my skin. I laughed to hide my embarrassment, but at that moment everything changed. Suddenly colour mattered, in more ways than one. This is when I realised I was black. It was like I had turned up to a party to which I was not invited. I felt irrelevant, excluded and ashamed. The message from the beauty industry was loud and clear: I was not valuable enough to be part of the conversation.'[2]

When I was young I would choose a foundation that was too light for my skin tone, trying to mimic the porcelain skin of the women who were celebrated as beautiful when I was growing up through the nineties. It was obvious, even from an early age, that wealth equated to a certain type of skin and hair and teeth, and that whiteness equated to beauty.

Beauty privilege is something appearance activist and disability advocate Carly Findlay knows a lot about. As she explained both in her ground-breaking memoir, *Say Hello*, and in her advocacy work, her lived experience as someone with facial difference means that she is constantly in receipt of scrutiny and discrimination due to her appearance. 'So while people with beauty privilege, people without facial differences or a disability, might have body image issues that stem from themselves or the way they see other people in the media or social media, I have had to put that behind. For me, there are a lot bigger issues to think about.'[3]

I became so accustomed to the way my face looked with makeup layered upon my skin that I have continued to do it almost the same way for decades. The idea that I might change the colour of my lipstick makes me panic. 'I wouldn't be me,' I fret.

The deep issues that this exposes in the way I relate to my body are not lost on me. We know through numerous studies that young women are suffering enormous psychological impacts from the pressures associated with living up to the ideals on display on social media platforms like Instagram and that mass marketing has forever preyed on our fears.[4] But we possibly don't speak enough about the pressure that women place on themselves and each other.

The attacks levelled at advocates like Melissa Blake attempt to ensure she is diminished and made small, and the controlling narratives about who is and isn't beautiful also sometimes come from the soldiers within our ranks. Women who have been advantaged by this system are also interested in maintaining the types of control that disadvantage others.

I met a woman at the pub a couple of years ago when I was first thinking about these questions of age. She had beautiful flowing grey hair and a petite figure. To my eyes, she looked glorious. Somehow we found ourselves in a discussion about age, and I told her that I was thinking of writing a book on the questions that I had about it. The air around us went cold, her eyes narrowed, and she looked me up and down. 'What would you know?' she derided. 'Do you dye your hair? Shave your legs? Still have sex?' I was so shocked by the questioning. The anger I felt at this judgement was overwhelming. 'Are you serious?' I asked, hoping she'd have a good reason to question me this way. She seemed excited to get a rise out of me, rubbing her hands together as she grilled me on my feminist responsibility to ageing, as if by allowing herself to go grey she had somehow pushed back. I didn't think she had.

We said a lot of things to each other about what we saw as the problems as women who were ageing. It became clear to me, speaking with her, that there was a crucial element to all of this. That without a cease-fire, an agreement to hold off on judgement of each other, we were enacting the plan of the patriarchy – we were doing the job of the system that we claimed to rail against. When we told each other how we were supposed to look, to age, to mother, to love, to be young girls – all of it – we destroyed ourselves.

It was the kind of exchange you can only have with a stranger. The sort of 'no rules' that can be difficult to navigate with friends you've had for thirty years. We had nothing to lose and so much to gain as we spoke. It was a moment a great exposition of what age can allow between people: a tender and kind disagreement of the most passionate variety. But then, in another, the exposure of great caverns of ideological space between us.

Her ideas to me seemed to enforce a fear we'd had for a long time: women just can't win. Women are either old and forgotten or, if they undertake any form of cosmetic procedures, are seen to have betrayed the sisterhood. This woman had been clearly celebrated for her ageing beauty but believed that she was in some way holding a hard line.

She worked as a lawyer and so her cachet, one could argue, was not harmed by her 'stately' demeanour. What was concerning to me was that she assumed an equal playing field for all women. The oldness that we despised didn't look like her. It was poverty and oldness, disability and oldness, coloured and oldness. And it was in these intersections that oldness became dangerous.

The conversation exposed that the white cis voice is so frequently centred in issues concerning women that we remain blind to the greater disparity of treatment. If you're a rich white woman, chances are your ageing can become yet another advantage because you have been able to do it 'well'. We cannot separate the ideal of beauty from privilege and a distortion and control of what is ultimately powerful. Possibly the main factor in accessing a beauty standard is privilege. How beautiful we are, how well we are able to maintain that beauty through our ageing, serves as an indicator of a class status, cultural coding and privilege.[5]

It doesn't seem like we should attribute a sense of personal achievement if ageing has been done in a highly controlled and enormously advantaged environment full of good food, exercise and affirming images of other thin white women proliferated through the media, but somehow it is still sold that way. Historically, conforming to beauty norms meant conforming to 'white' beauty norms. 'The most common cosmetic operations requested before the 20th century aimed to correct features such as ears, noses and breasts classified as "ugly" because they weren't typical for "white" people.'[6]

Where once cosmetic surgery and cosmetic procedures were solely the realm of the rich and famous, they now belong to the cultures of the middle and lower classes: filling, sucking, cutting, sculpting, tucking, plucking, colouring and needling. For many decades women have hidden the changes that were made to their bodies. If surgery happened, it was done in secret. It was imperative that no one should think beauty was accessed unnaturally.

Since at least the 1950s, women have overwhelmingly been the target consumers for cosmetic surgery, while men have practised it: males represented 85.9 per cent of clinicians in 2016 and had an average age of 52.7 years. Women represented 14.1 per cent of clinicians and were on average 5.4 years younger than male clinicians.[7]

And while modern cosmetic surgery and procedures rely upon mass marketing and social media to provide fertile opportunities for women to feel inadequate, cosmetic surgery has dated back to the availability of anaesthesia that allowed for a painless procedure.[8]

Around the turn of the twentieth century, advertisements spruiked contraptions to aid in the preservation or return of youth. Professor Eugene Mack of 507 Fifth Avenue in New York City offered a mechanism that could give the 'Curves of Youth' if you just 'Pull the Cords'. The mechanism looks medieval, attaching around the face with straps and cords and promising to produce a 'concentrated, continuous massage of the chin and neck, dispelling flabbiness of the neck and throat, restoring a rounded contour to thin, scrawny necks and faces, bringing a natural, healthy color to the cheeks, effacing lines and wrinkles. Price only $10.'[9]

In the modern era, while we accept cosmetic interventions, these procedures and the women who undertake them are policed. Some women know to look above the lips of conspicuous women to see if there are any pinholes. Are those lips injected? Surely they are not natural? She's paid for them – she must have. Women I know talk about when the work has gone beyond the threshold of what we collectively agree is acceptable. 'She's gone too far,' is what is whispered 'Her lips are way too full. Her forehead is way too smooth.'

There seems to be a macabre delight when we see that women have gone too far. When this cosmetic advantage becomes something to laugh at or feel superior to. We are scorned when we age, or ignored, but if we try to avoid the social shaming of age by paying for fillers or peels or surgery, we are thought of as if we have cheated.

The homogenous definition of femininity is not simply inflicted by a commercial agenda – there is also judgement that is unleashed on women, by women. There are powerful agendas perpetrated by the elite classes to ensure the exclusion of certain women. How we are controlled is done by ourselves.

There is a significant class dimension to how our 'age defying' is policed. If women have access to healthy food, clean water, dental hygiene, exercise and a manageable workload, their chances of ageing 'well' are obviously increased. What happens when poor women are also able to access beauty products and cosmetic services that will enable them to look acceptable as they age? It seems that now, with access to these procedures for more strata of class and culture, the script is being flipped on which age-defying work is acceptable.

We have shifted towards a narrative that sees some cosmetic procedures as a low-status activity while ageing 'gracefully' is seen as high. When women in lower socio-economic brackets cannot access value via other modes of capital then it might be possible to accrue value through beauty itself.[10]

While acceptance and access has enabled individuals to undertake various forms of cosmetic procedures, there remains a class divide in how the corrections are viewed more broadly. The rise in eyelash extensions, a relatively affordable enhancement, has been enthusiastically embraced by young women. The appeal of eyelash extensions has many theories, including that long eyelashes are valuable for the fact that they create the illusion of the wide, gazing eyes and therefore supports ideas we have about a young face eliciting a desire to protect.[11] But the access to this eyelash procedure and the extent to which it has been embraced, not to mention the length to which these lashes have literally grown, has relegated the procedure to the cultural and economic lower classes.

The way we have responded to increases in cosmetic procedures and the types that are able to be accessed has been about ensuring non-white, poor and disabled women are kept at a disadvantage. Perhaps the undercurrent here is far more insidious: if poor women can access the same advantage that has historically only been the privilege of the rich, then the 'advantage' no longer exists. It loses its currency.

* * *

Justine Bateman took a punk attitude to her ageing face. Once the good-looking, girl-next-door teen in the hit eighties sitcom *Family Ties*, she wrote a book interrogating the cultural norms around ageing. In a discussion with *Vanity Fair* about her book, she acknowledges the ubiquity of plastic surgery going from '"Wow, that plastic surgery is so extreme" to "When are you getting your plastic surgery?" ... It's almost your duty now as a [woman] to start cutting up your face.'[12]

But what does it mean to look young? What are the dimensions of youth? How is this sold to us so that not only do we pay for it but are coerced to undertake it in secret? The anti-ageing industry is continuing to see enormous growth. In 2019, Australian women were spending $7.1 billion a year on beauty with a significant proportion of the pie allocated to women who wanted to look more youthful.[13]

Anti-ageism activist Ashton Applewhite, author of *This Chair Rocks: A Manifesto Against Ageism*, pointed out in a discussion with Katie Couric on her podcast that 'if ageing is framed as a problem, we can be persuaded to buy stuff to "fix it" or "stop it" ... you can't make money off satisfaction. So there's a multibillion-dollar anti-ageing skin-care industry, a trillion-dollar pharmaceutical industry that says, 'Oh, if you can't remember the name of that movie you saw, you have mild cognitive impairment and you'd better buy this game or take this drug.'"[14]

Applewhite sees the need for a grassroots movement against ageism in all its forms. To rise up and call it out. To make changes in how we teach young people to understand age. She argues that we need to stop medicalising ageing and push back against unhelpful and unfounded stereotypes of the ageing experience.

* * *

The question many of us are still asking is whether cosmetic procedures are empowering self-actualisation or a capitulation to the capitalist system that built us to know ourselves as lacking. Am I a bad feminist if I get a bit of Botox here and there? If I know that my response has been influenced by systemic oppression but I want to do it anyway?

A new generation of women is pushing back and attempting to change the value we place on cosmetic procedures. Women more empowered now with access to their own wealth are demanding their changed bodies are seen through the prism of their success. That they have earned their beauty rather than been unfairly born with it.

Some women are demanding that they are proud of the adjustments that they have made to their bodies because for some younger people it is a sign of emancipation. They have earned their own freedom. It is a sense that, regardless of how or why we are incarcerated, at least we have choice in how we navigate this incarceration.

The move by young women towards 'body positivity as empowerment' has also promoted the idea that a changed face can be empowering. Young people are not only making 'corrections' to their faces but also alterations. A plastic surgery website that I stumbled across was using the intersection of empowerment and the changed self to its advantage under a headline that read 'The Normalisation of Plastic Surgery – Don't be Ashamed of Your Cosmetic Surgeries'. The empowerment that was being claimed by women was being harnessed and used against them on this plastic surgery site: 'Celebrities like Iggy Azalea owning up to their surgeries and proudly admitting them helps the average woman to have realistic expectations for their bodies. It also gives them the courage to do something about things they don't like … The real benefit in the changing attitudes toward plastic surgery is the chance for women and men to take control of their bodies. If you love your natural breasts … great! If you don't, change them. Plastic surgery isn't an all or nothing proposition. It's an opportunity for us to sculpt our best selves. Natural or enhanced, there's no reason not to love your body.'[15]

But there is a cost to the normalisation of our changing faces. If changing your older face to embrace the features of youth becomes normalised, who will age? Who is going to look old? Who will be prepared to suffer a decrease in income when studies have shown that your 'attractiveness' (insert 'youthfulness') can achieve on average a twenty per cent increase in salary?[16] When face altering is normalised, what happens when you are the only one who doesn't participate?

Who will dare risk showing the world or other women or our children that looking old is not something we should fear? That oldness is a power? Or that we might look forward to the way age makes us look? When viewed through this prism, ageing naturally seems like an act of subversion. If we continue down the pathway that insists we must alter our faces and remain young, who will be our older generation? Who will cast that image of woman and stand up for her? Love her even?

ELEMENT:

Water

Parched

Water

Introduction

IT WAS ONLY ONE month after the Ash Wednesday fires tore through lives and land that the rain fell heavy from the sky. There had been drought here before, when livestock, in desperation and the madness of starvation, ate the dry earth in an attempt to fill their bellies.

When a drought creeps in and makes itself at home, it feels as if it will never leave. You believe that this is the way you are going to die.

When those rains fell in March 1983, they didn't stop. It is how droughts often work. Long periods of life-changing thirst, and then the rain falls like it had never stopped. 'Why were you worried, silly girl? There was always going to be rain. You think I would leave you here to die?'

Over the next twelve months there was more rain than usual, 822 millimetres filling dams and quenching the earth. It felt as though water had the power to wash away any memory we might have had of our desperate thirst. Once thirst is quenched, it's difficult to remember what it feels like to hunger for it. Once your thirst disappears, you can't quite recall why it felt so terrible.

The land had been brown and hard for so long that many had forgotten it could be any other way. Unlike fire, there is no one moment of trauma during a drought, just a prolonged torture. Soon, though, after the rains came, the landscape returned to green, and the dams filled. And it almost seemed like nothing had ever happened. You could be forgiven for believing it had always been this way, lush and full of love.

* * *

I have understood that strange, frantic desire for water. I know what it feels like to thirst for it, when your body is screaming for it, dreaming to be drowned in it. I have wanted to drink it up so that I might be overflowing. I know what it feels like to want for it so single-mindedly that you can think of nothing else. And my desire to be so full of it that water spills out of me, staining my shirt, consuming every part of me – that I might feel it run cold through every tributary.

I was in my mid-twenties and had found myself again in hospital. By this stage, it had been weeks. I had come out of surgery that had attached an ileostomy bag a few days before, but now my bowel had twisted and was obstructed. Nothing would go down. I had vomited every last drop of liquid from my body – my earth was parched, and it took every inch of me to attempt to try to deal with the pain of thirst.

It was vicious and I was maddened by its unrelenting cry. I had already come to understand that in this sort of pain, you must find a way to stop fighting. I had learnt through other bouts of relentless pain that I needed to find the strength to lie still, to allow it to cover me. I realised the fight I was trying to put up wasn't going to save me. And so I prayed that something would make me sleep or otherwise render me unconscious.

A couple of years earlier, I had been diagnosed with Crohn's disease. What had started out as an illness I thought I might manage with medication soon became a condition that took me to bed for years. By that time in hospital, I had lost everything I had thought mattered to me: university, my house, work, my independence. And I was forced to understand earlier than most that our bodies will ultimately betray us. Even before we become old, some of us understand that this body will break and ultimately dictate the kind of experience we will have as 'human'.

That particular day, lying in that hospital bed by myself, it had felt like I was made only of matter and bones. I wasn't my dreams or my imagination. Instead, the pain demanded that I be lodged deep inside the experience of my body. I was too terrified to leave it and drift away in case it consumed me whole while I was somewhere else. I hungered so much to drink that I willed water to break through my skin, like it does when it hits the earth and seeps down, down, and then transforms itself into its host – becoming the earth, damp and alive.

I finally drifted off to sleep and dreamt of the time when I was five years old and I was taught how to swim. The excitement of bathers sticking to skin when the water nourishes you all over. I loved diving into that quiet world beneath the surface, below sound, where everything is both dulled and magnified. A place I could be alone with my thoughts. 'Blow out,' they said. 'Blow bubbles under the water.' I smiled at the other children who were blowing bubbles and put my head under, blowing the biggest bubbles I could. My world filled my ears and I could hear my voice bubbling.

In my childish arrogance, I thought they were teaching us about bubble blowing so that we understood not to breathe under water. I just assumed that the other children didn't get this basic concept, and this was just another one of those lessons you are given as a child with the heading 'How to survive as a human being'. I thought we were being taught this so we wouldn't confuse ourselves with fish. Lesson: we were human, and we didn't really belong in the water.

So I never learnt to swim. I spent the first thirty years of my life not blowing bubbles when I swam and instead held my breath until I couldn't hold it any longer. It took one of my children, much later, to show me how to do it. 'Blow bubbles,' she said, laughing at me. 'Blow bubbles under the water, you idiot.'

* * *

In the city, the 1982 drought meant we needed to change the way we understood water. Before the drought I played under the sprinkler on those nights when the air was thick and still and hot, and we knew we wouldn't be able to sleep. It was a time before we had air conditioners or passive housing. We would turn on the tap for hours and let the water run over our hot bodies. There was a clown sprinkler whose hat flew into the air when the water pumped through the hose.

Soon we would be on water rations, timing the length of our showers with no more lazy weekends washing the car and a schedule for when we could water our gardens, odd-numbered houses on certain days, even on the others. Our next-door neighbours ran their water on the days they weren't supposed to and what was once a friendly relationship became tinged with suspicion and resentment that lasted another twenty years. 'Why do they think they can water their gardens when the rest of the bloody country can't?' the neighbourhood would whisper over fences and around kitchen tables.

* * *

Water is a shape-shifter, fluid and transitional. It will become whatever it needs to be. It is also the greatest of diplomats as it belongs to both the earth and sky. But like fire, it has no regard for life when it seeks its own desires. It is ferocious when it wants to be and shows its power without hesitation. And while it can rumble as loud as any natural disaster with a tsunami or flood, it can also be deathly silent, denying the world its essence as the earth and every living thing upon it dies.

Ageing was beginning to feel like a deep fatigue resting inside my bones. And I knew that it would be easier, much easier, to stay in bed. I wanted to feel like I had as a child when I would push my head down, submerged in the Harold Holt pool, and all I could hear were the muffled sounds of life around me. I wanted to swim down to where I could hide away from the world outside.

I knew I had to try to resist the fight. To accept the pain that a drought would bring me with the full knowledge that water may never return to my spring. That this is perhaps how I was going to die.

It felt, as I was confronted by the changing shape of water, that I had to learn to lie still, to stop fighting and float above the tumult. When I was a little girl it was my greatest skill in the water. Perhaps my only one. I would fill my lungs and launch my body to float above the water. I would push my head back and lift my chest to the sky. And I would float for stretches of time that made it feel that when I returned to standing, the world around me was now completely different.

* * *

I could see the change in me reflected in the water. Going back through human history, water was once the only way we could see ourselves, reflected in its disjointed mirror.

Like Narcissus, we are enamoured and tortured by our reflection. When Narcissus was a child, a prophecy was made by a blind seer that he would live a long and happy life if he did not know himself. Perhaps what she saw was a prophecy for all of us. How much do we lose of ourselves when we look at our reflection? What sort of stories do we tell ourselves about our age simply because we have looked rather than felt?

And like water, there is a world of truth that lives below that surface of us and is more complex to find. Water rushes through our worlds inside and outside us. The surface of our planet is seventy-one per cent water while our own bodies are sixty per cent, and we feel the tug of the tides as they ebb and recede inside us.

This is the part of the story of ageing where we reckon with the trauma of our bodies, sharing our secrets with each other when they become too painful to continue to give refuge. The water is where we face the loss and the love that we have experienced, the amniotic fluid that breaks and is unleashed all over the kitchen floor. It is a birthing. And a death.

Water

CHAPTER 10

Under Water: Secrets

DEEP IN THE OCEAN, fish speak to each other. We didn't know this for the longest time. We imagined they communicated with colour and body and electricity. But now scientists have found that they are like birds, and they have a dusk and a dawn chorus. It was just that for a long time we didn't hear them. In fact, fish have spoken for something like 155 million years, and it's just now that we've learnt how we might need to listen.[1]

The world that lives inside the waters on earth is a mystery. It is unsurprising that our oceans are the most unexplored and unknown parts of the entire planet. We know only a mere twentieth of their totality. The rest is an unmapped mystery.

* * *

When I was fifteen, I had a best friend. When I saw her, I felt as if I was looking in a kind of mirror and seeing something of myself, a self that lived in an entirely different body. She was exciting. She enjoyed playing with danger. I watched her as she often almost teetered over the edge.

Sometimes all we would need to do was speak to each other with our eyes, the smallest of movements. It was as if words had passed between us. I wondered if somehow we had breathed words to each other through a special slipstream, one that you can only access with someone who feels like they are you. We would spend hours together when hardly anything would be said. When you've reached that stage of knowing, words are often not helpful.

That sort of friendship is a kind of first love. Platonic and simple, it's built on how it feels to be near each other and how it feels to be seen. We had learnt to read each other like a weather system and could see a change from kilometres away and adjust and prepare accordingly. Pull in the sails, the storm will be big, and our laughter would roll around each other like thunder, twisting and climbing into the sky.

I have known other people like this in my life. The way you know and love each other means you can break down the space that lives to separate you. You glide effortlessly between living inside each other and living outside. And sometimes it's hard to know where you are because it begins to feel so much like the same. When you spend that amount of time in someone else's space, you learn to hear a quickening of breath, a change in tone. You know an awful lot without speaking.

We would share secrets with each other. Every secret. There was nothing between our skin that we hadn't shared. It is beautiful to know that your secrets can also be held inside someone else. That someone else can take part of them for you. It is a power to know that a secret is special enough to be housed somewhere as precious as your best friend. And the trust you have for them to house it is as precious as gold.

After several wild years in each other's lives, we eventually drifted apart. She moved interstate and I haven't seen her for a couple of decades now. She took my secrets with her, the ones that I had held close to me all those years ago. The ones that belonged to me when I had the body of a teenager. I am still holding some of hers that are now just a flutter, a feeling deep inside me. Secrets that made me cry when I first heard them and are now awash with everything that has come since. But they are there, and I could find them if she needed me to.

But some secrets could never be shared because we simply didn't know we had been housing them. That we had been holding them deep inside us for the women who had travelled this earth thousands of years before. By virtue of being women, there are secrets that are trapped inside that have been carried through our blood for an age. We carry the trauma of our gendered experience just underneath our skin. And depending on our skill, we can keep that trauma down deep inside. If we are not so skilled, we might notice the trauma because those secrets well up and become bright red boils on top of our skin. It is the wildness that visits us with the moon.

* * *

Secrets are built on the foundation of a kind of shame. Or sometimes because we know that no one can be trusted to take the kind of care that the secret needs. And as we age, it seems harder and harder to prise those secrets from where they calcified onto our bones. How do you speak of something that now cannot be pulled apart from the person that you have become? Your secrets, your shame, soon become a solid part of you. It is the quiet rumblings in the middle of the night that remind you that you are not someone who should be loved.

Do you remember going to the beach as a kid and burying yourself deep in the sand? Hours and hours it would take to dig those holes with our tiny hands until they were big enough to lower our little bodies inside. And then we would beg for someone to trap us inside by filling the hole back in. The enormous weight of the sand making it impossible to move our bodies free.

But this is how we liked it. We couldn't move, so no one could blame us if we didn't. And in just the same way, we treated our secrets like this. No one expected to hear them, so we didn't have a choice about these secrets. No one should blame us if we kept quiet. This was enforced silence. We had been paid off.

Sharing secrets was something we intuitively knew we shouldn't do, because those secrets were often about how we had fallen. How we had been coerced into violence. How our private selves had been violated and would continue to be violated were we to bring it up in public. Best to keep it quiet is what we all learnt.

Shame keeps our secrets locked in place. That is, until someone scrapes around the line of your body and you can wriggle yourself free. First it's your little finger, and then it's your whole arm. When your secrets find their way free, sometimes it can feel as if you are transitioning from immovable to weightless. When the first whispers of the secret are finally set free, it feels as if the darkness that has inhabited you is also momentarily free.

Women are good at keeping secrets. We are good at silence, at keeping our heads down and pretending not to see. We know what will happen if we are complicit in the crimes. We know how to avoid that sort of responsibility. It's easy for us, too, if we believe what we've been told. Only sluts get themselves into trouble, the girls wearing the wrong thing late at night. What do they expect?

Giving away the secrets of perpetrators can sometimes cost us our place at the table. Easier to assert that it's not something that would happen to the good women. Just the fast ones. The loose ones. The ones who were asking for it.

Or the coloured or disabled or fat girls who don't know their place. We know what happens to them if they dare think they're more than what they've been told they are. They are laughed at for trying to keep up. For trying to behave as if they too deserve the same kind of love.

The crimes that eventually stir us into rage are when the pretty girls are attacked in places that we might find ourselves. Or our daughters. Or the girls who are pure. We recognise violence only sometimes. Other times we expect it; we've learnt that when you're not what they want, you deserve it.

We have kept secrets, trapped inside our thin lips, that we hold on to at all costs. We keep these secrets to protect ourselves against the destruction that we know awaits us if, somehow, we think ourselves brave enough to speak up. We grew up with the 'keep quiet or else' mantra and we saw what happened to the ones who thought they could get away with talking back.

* * *

We have seen it time and time again. When women stand up to tell their stories of sexual assault, it is their version of events put under the microscope. What was she wearing? Had she been drinking? How had she been behaving at work to send such mixed messages? We knew that these sorts of 'transgressions' could lead to a woman getting hurt, and we came to understand that they could happen on the streets and in our homes. The rough handling of women, the raping, the killing – we had become accustomed to expect there was danger out there.

But to accept that these sorts of crimes might be committed in our workplaces was unthinkable. To imagine that in these pristine environments of suits and ties and office desks and memos, that such violence could take place, is much harder to fathom and therefore much harder to believe.

Unsurprisingly, there is an unwillingness to come forward when sexual harassment has been experienced in the workplace. The Australian Human Rights Commission, led by Kate Jenkins, the Sexual Discrimination Commissioner, released the Respect@Work report in March 2020. The 18-month inquiry into sexual harassment in Australian workplaces exposed that while over a third of workers recorded sexual harassment while only 17% had made a complaint.[2]

So, what causes someone to finally speak after having their head pushed into the dirt? 'Shhh,' they hiss, 'no point making a noise; they'll just think you're lying.' What compels a woman into known danger to tell the stories we've all been told are the ones we must keep to ourselves at all costs? You'll get hurt. You know you will. So why do it?

Many have suggested that the motivation for women to disclose violence in workplaces is to enact revenge. In fact, four in ten Australians believe sexual assault accusations are a way of getting back at men.[3] They must be the fictions of disgruntled women who didn't get their way, is the perception. The theory is that women have extraordinary power and interest to lie about the behaviour of men for their own advantage. The problem with this thesis is that the advantage that is assumed is well documented not to exist. In fact, an overwhelming majority of women don't report sexual assault at all, as the system has failed to protect women who have gone before them. Human rights lawyer and Kurin MinangNoongar woman Dr Hannah McGlade cites research that shows many victims will never make it to a police station, 'and this is particularly true for Indigenous women ... Aboriginal women may not report for multiple reasons, including fear of the perpetrator, fear of being in a small community and lack of faith in the police.'[4]

You find out, often too late, that it's an under-resourced and ill-equipped bureaucracy that will hear your story. It is a system with a default setting of 'lying whore'. It is your responsibility to prove otherwise. We see it time and time again when sexual assault stories make their way to the courts and women are ripped to shreds to infer their complicit behaviour or inherent seduction is at the root of why they were attacked. It's obvious by what she was wearing that she was asking for it. Why would she have gone behind the shed with those two men otherwise? 'Come get me, boys' was what she had been implying.

Everyone knew it.

Nadia was the woman who was taken behind a shed at a party in regional Victoria in 2017 and who reported the alleged rape by two older men. Eventually, her case against these two men went to trial.[5]

The way Nadia was questioned by the defence barristers

during the first of two trials has become an issue of scrutiny. The ABC reported that 'Legal experts, criminologists and mental health workers have all raised concerns about what these transcripts show. One criminologist says the questions that two defence barristers asked Nadia during the first trial should "shock our moral consciousness".

> **Barrister 1:** And what were you wearing?
> **Nadia:** I was wearing boots, jeans, a belt, a leather jacket, a jumper underneath, and a top underneath that.
> **Barrister 1:** Was the top underneath that a – can you describe the top that was underneath the—?
> **Nadia:** It was long-sleeved, and high neckline, black.
> **Barrister 1:** And what sort of material was it made out of?
> **Nadia:** Sheer material.

The other defence barrister went further with his cross-examination.

> **Barrister 2:** You took the jumper off at an early stage of the evening, is that right?
> **Nadia:** Yes, and I was still wearing my jacket.
> **Barrister 2:** So your jacket and a sheer shirt that I think people have described as being see-through, so you had like some kind of under – a bra or something under that?
> **Nadia:** I have something over my bra, but under my shirt, yes.
> **Barrister 2:** So when yesterday you just said you were wearing a jumper, was that to downplay the actual state of your dress that night?[6]

Later in the first trial, it was a comment made by a judge about Nadia's virginity that also shocked and traumatised Nadia. He said, 'It strikes me as being relevant to an issue as to whether a seventeen-year-old girl who's had no experience of intercourse at all before would choose to break her duck, so to speak, with two men, vaginal, anal and oral, on the ground, in the dark.' The reference to 'break her duck' is about the first time you score a run in a cricket match and a reference to Nadia's virginity.

It feels as if the legal system is set up to expose what the system has always believed to be the truth: sluts are asking for it, look at what she was wearing.

* * *

A few brave women have lifted up their heads, knowing they would be punished, to pierce the very centre of that silence and raise their voices to tell the truth about what it is like to live as a woman. They tell a story that reflects our own – of being forced to dance the dangerous line between purity and desire even at work, while trying to get by and remain safe.

In 2020, a grief was awoken in us. After hearing the stories that emerged about sexual harrassment at work with the Respect@Work report and having spent years now holding vigil for the women who had been killed on our streets and in our homes, an enormous rage seemed to take hold that suddenly felt impossible to hold down. Women were horrified to hear their own stories being told back to us this way. The details were different, but the song was the same. We had all learnt to hum along with that tune.

It brought into stark relief the enormous pain and the humiliation of it all, that women had dared to be considered in the same realm as men. So embedded is the misogyny that we barely understand how to recognise it. We are constantly flicking the rubber band on our wrist trying to remember 'it's not her fault' while harbouring years and years of teachings that say the opposite. Hasn't it always been the bad girls who find themselves in bad situations? And surely there's got to be some truth to that?

What we've been convinced to believe is that it was common for women to give off all the wrong sorts of signals. Only certain sorts of women are to be regarded with the kind of respect that would mean that they weren't to blame.

We felt the searing humiliation of this abuse. To remember ourselves as young girls with the hopes that one day we might be loved and valued for the ferocious minds and hearts that beat inside us, but come to understand that our dreams can be used against us. We were filled with excitement that we might one day be someone of worth, beyond the catcalls and whistles. Then we found it was just play, that we would never be considered as good as the boys. It was all just a game that they allowed us to believe we might have a chance at winning until they got us alone and could have us the way they really wanted us.

And when we hear the testimony of those women, our own stories rise from inside us, lying long dormant in a darkness that has become so familiar we had stopped noticing it. Emerging to sit just at the top of our skin so that if we were bumped at all we'd start to bleed.

As we age, those secrets, so hardened on our bones, can somehow be knocked loose and find their way out of us. Like a parasite that has devoured all the available flesh and now needs to find its way to another host. There becomes little option but to spill the darkness on the floor, to release it somehow.

During those weeks that surrounded the March4Justice, I found it hard to listen to people – who believed they had a specific right to a voice simply because they were women – when they declared this wasn't their lived experience. The 'woke' men who have long protested that it's not them who perpetrate the violence against women. The sad eyes of faux understanding for what it has been like to sit on the other side of the table to women.

The men who are convinced that they have not been taught to hate women are the ones to watch out for most because their misogyny is not understood by them. In fact, they have built an identity that strives to distance themselves from the very thought that they might have also been taught that some women probably deserve it.

For me, the most dangerous men became the ones who believed that this wasn't about them. The men who thought that they were on our side, who believed that they would never debase a woman like this. These were the men who assumed that they had been immune to the way we had all been taught to know women as less. Not me, they would say, I love women.

We have been coerced into keeping these secrets. To not tell young girls entering the space of women about the horrors we've experienced. To only whisper them to each other, and only when we trust that the stories won't be used against us.

We've been taught that we cannot use the justice system or raise our voices in public domains because the system maintains its power by eradicating anyone who tries to rattle it. It happens time and time again. There is no room to heal the hurt, we must just get rid of them at all costs.

Are we afraid to tell our children of this world because we worry it will somehow invoke a similar fate? Do we not want them to know that we have been tarnished? Soiled and disgraced? Is it the continuum of shame that keeps us quiet? The knowledge that you must have somehow been responsible?

And then what? How do we reconcile the secrets that we have kept for so long in these old bodies? In a world that hasn't changed, that is still wondering how to view a woman who has been raped and how to deal with the men who perpetrate rape — where do we take this experience and how do we understand it?

How do we age with this inside us?

* * *

I have hidden my own secrets and kept my own silence. Many times. As have my friends.

When I was growing up, there was an unspoken understanding that any violence you encountered was likely because you had done something you shouldn't have. Always masked in a faux understanding that you had been hurt, but moments later you became very aware that the weight of blame would be placed on you. It would always circle back to you like a homing pigeon. There was no escaping that you were responsible.

One of my good friends had been seeing a psychiatrist for one of the abuses she experienced in her early twenties. She told him about the circumstances of what happened to her: she vaguely knew the boy, had been speaking to him at a party.

That night, while she was sleeping in the lounge room after everyone had gone home, she woke up with him on top of her. When she went through the details of the assault, the psychiatrist looked at her like she was an idiot. He pointed out the window of his office to where men in hi-vis were doing roadwork.

'You see those holes?' he said, trying to help her see what was obvious to him with a simple metaphor that she might understand.

'Yes,' she nodded warily, already sensing that she had divulged this secret to a man who was going to use it against her.

'Well, if you go outside and walk around those holes and you fall in ...' He looked at her, hoping her simple brain might understand what he was trying to get at. 'Well, if you fall in, do you think you might have known that it was dangerous?'

She looked at him, rage making its way out of her in tears that were now spilling.

'He looked bewildered,' she told me. 'I think he must have thought that telling me it was my fault that I had been raped must have been hard for me to hear.'

But no matter how much she knew in her heart that he was wrong, something inside her believed it too. She knew it wasn't right, not by the letter of the law, because clearly people shouldn't do that to each other, but she still wonders if her signals were all wrong. Had she been responsive in her sleep somehow?

We keep our silence for so many reasons. Sometimes it's because we don't believe anyone will care, or that somehow it must have been our fault. Or that we have no energy to hope for understanding or love from those who have the power to protect us. When we are so deeply embedded with the shame of these bodies, it's difficult to feel empowered to understand that this is not inherently our fault.

* * *

I walked through Treasury Gardens in Melbourne in 2020 on a day, somewhere in the middle of a pandemic, when we gathered to remember the women who had died at the hands of violence and the women who had been subjected to physical and mental abuse. It was a march for women. We had done these kinds of walks before.

When I was in my twenties, I would go alone to the Reclaim the Night protests and dance to the drumbeats and shouts of freedom from the women. I would fill myself with them and be lost in the excitement. The air was fresh and it hummed, like those first moments of spring when there is a wildness in the way it feels to have your skin brushed by warm breezes. We walked with each other like we shared skin. We didn't have to say anything because we all knew what it was like to walk around as women. These marches were a way to assert an idea of some sort of freedom.

In the nineties, my teenage years, women explored their identities through anti-fashion and 'masculine' expressions of femininity – army boots, flannelettes, ripped jeans, and makeup that had been applied to highlight the absurdity, overwhelming eyes with black lines to expose the folly.

But I didn't really believe that women could be free. I didn't have faith that there might be a world where women's bodies were safe. Of course, it was something we spoke about, but we knew we were powerless to ever make it a reality. Because ultimately, it was still our fault if we were out at night and got hurt. It was still our fault if we dressed in a way that had made a man unable to control his violence against us. When I was in my twenties, these marches were just a way to say that it wasn't okay without any real hope that anything would ever change.

The feeling of marching together when I was young was more a sense of joy at the rebelliousness of the congregation, the power in being surrounded by other women. No one could hurt us here; we had each other as shields. We could disappear into an ocean of women and be free. No one would be looking at just me because there were too many of us and in every iteration. There was a shared experience of what it was to identify as a woman and have that hang around us like a noose. I felt free there. I still can feel that inside me, the velvet of my skirt against my skin.

But in 2020, the march was different. It felt like the joy of rebellion had been replaced by a desperate knowing that nothing had changed, that nothing might ever change, and we had been seriously hurt. We had been killed.

Women were streaming in from trams and trains. There was a deafening silence. A shared understanding that we had gathered to do a job. It was not built on rage this time. It felt more like a deep and abiding grief. A depth of sorrow for the loss. A rawness for how the violence left our skin exposed.

In Treasury Gardens, we bore witness to a scroll with the names of 899 women and children who had been killed since 2008. Women and children who had been killed in their homes by the men they had at one time trusted, whom they once loved. There was a collective knowing of the pain. The searing humiliation. The ache in our guts for the children killed or hurt or forever scarred.

I have never felt anything like it before. A tremendous love enveloping us all. A trusted space to finally look up and into each other's eyes. 'You too?' they would say without words. 'Yes, me too,' would be the answer. And a love and knowing would flow between us. 'I am here.'

We are trapped in this system of violence. It is a language that so many of us have learnt to speak. When one of us dies, it is a grief that we feel inside for all of us. For the families, for the community, for our dumb ways of doing things.

When the study was launched, The 2018 Australian Trans and Gender Diverse Sexual Health Survey recruited the largest sample of trans and gender-diverse people to an Australian research study. The survey found that transgender women were four times more likely to experience sexual coercion and/or violence than the general Australian public. What is additionally concerning with these figures is that transgender women who seek care and support related to their sexual health and safety experience marginalisation due to their gender. The women who most need support are the least likely to access it and find access to it safely.[7]

* * *

For the first time, women were speaking openly about their own experiences of abuse. It wasn't 'if' you had experienced sexual assault but rather when and how. I was working in radio that day and had run from the studio to be there. I had a microphone in my hand and was able to access the stories of women in a way that is not normally available. The microphone can become a portal for using our voices to make them loud.

Sometimes the microphone can be a way to whisper secrets that we know we need to share.

What shocked me was how widespread the abuse must be. We had been through this before when #metoo erupted around the world in 2017. But there was something different about this. Something quieter, more personal. Something that fuelled a grief and a rage like I hadn't seen in this country before.

That day, it felt as if everything was done in a whisper. That the secrets that had been black inside us had to find a way out of us, but quietly at first. Because there is so much shame in those first moments of revelation.

Most women I reached with my microphone had been crying. Many women had come with the various generations that made up their families. Young girls, teenagers, mothers, grandmothers were here together, crying about the life that we were all living or had lived.

There were survivors with placards describing how they had escaped with their lives, but only just. They still bore scars that would likely never leave them.

This wasn't a march where we cheered and screamed into the night, the smoke of our battle fires burning for all to see. This time it was about the grief we collectively feel when we have lost someone. When we have lost something. When we are lost women.

And it felt like there was a realisation that there is no way back. We'd crossed over into the space where if we don't make this new, if we don't find a way to change this for our young girls, we will continue to die. It felt exhausting, like we had hit a wall, and it was the same wall we'd been hitting for generations.

Was this about the compounding trauma of the systemic and cultural issues that women continued to face? Every year it seemed we had taken to the streets after a woman had been violently murdered or had shaken our heads at the rise in domestic violence and the deaths of women in their own homes. And each time it felt like the emotions were hotter. The temperature higher. One year in Melbourne it felt as if we were visiting, on a regular basis, the crime scenes of women who had been murdered, all of us in tears for a woman we hadn't known but felt we had through the way we can know ourselves in each other.

I had been to most of the vigils. I felt I had a responsibility to be there. To bear witness. To see for myself. To see the grief of families. To stand in the same place that she had been only hours or days before and imagine what it must have been like to be her, suddenly grabbed and thrown to the ground. Many of us knew that feeling, but we hadn't been killed. Could we feel her here, in the air? How long would we think of her? How long would we share the memories of these women?

This wasn't about the rich and powerful men who had abused their status to sexually abuse women, this was about regular men who had abused their regular status to sexually abuse and humiliate women. This was about our silence. This was about how we had kept their secrets and how we continue to keep their secrets. This was about the wild and rampant grief and the amount of rage that was sitting just below our skin.

Getting older means carrying the burden of walking around in the image of women for years. And the landscape that changes as your form changes means that the resistance you may have built to endure it is suddenly transformed by the way your body codes. Sometimes it's those changes that open up the wounds that we've long tried to cover.

To be viewed differently in the world from how you were viewed only years before can clarify how you've been treated. To become suddenly invisible is the way we can understand how we have been seen for so long. The amount of power it has always held and the life that it created for us that we were too inside to see.

And with that change comes the rage of understanding the real cost of the burden of our bodies. The humiliation of them. The jokes that must be made about them when we're not in the room. When we've been forced out by powerful men who say that a woman's place is not at the table of power.

And if she makes her way there, we'll kill her, one way or another.

Water

CHAPTER 11

Currents: Blood

THAT BURNING FEELING WHEN I would tumble across the asphalt in the playground and sit up, trying not to cry, to find that my knees were full of small rubble and there was thick red blood dripping from them. Blood had always reminded me that we were fragile. That we could be opened up, and our insides could escape.

After scraping the dirt from the graze, I would secretly suck on the blood. It felt like I was breaking some unspoken rule, but there was a compulsion to do it. It tasted so good.

* * *

When I first started to bleed, I was humiliated. I looked in horror at the toilet paper. Blood had appeared from somewhere inside me without any warning. I had, I guess, expected more fanfare. Was this what it was, the first sign of this secret world that I'd heard so much about? Was this what I had been waiting anxiously for, this horror show of blood oozing from my body?

One of the ways that teachers tried to break down the divide between their world and our pre-pubescent lives was to attempt to 'speak the truth'. 'It's awful,' they would tell us, with feigned familiarity, like we were just a bunch of girls hanging out together at a sleepover. 'It's a drag,' they would say, flipping their eighties hairdos.

There was something that revolted me about this intimate world. Something unsettling and forced. A time in the movement when we knew we should be claiming this process, but we'd grown up with such a deeply embedded detestation for them that it was still just an act.

I had heard it would be difficult to deal with this every single month for the rest of my life and that it would hurt. I also knew I had to keep it secret. That was the deal – your period was a secret to be kept at all costs. And that secret-keeping was just another way to tell us that it was shame that we were dealing with.

But this bright red blood seemed so difficult to hide and so related to danger. It was coming out of me in a way that felt terrible. What did it mean to bleed like this? Beyond the physiology that we had been taught in health classes in school, it was also a symbol of our new-found vulnerability. We were officially people who menstruated. And while I had been intersecting in this world for some time, there was now no escape.

I recognised that I had crossed into something I had heard about for such a long time. By the definition of some, I was now a woman. And while it frightened me, it also held a mythical power. This type of womanhood was something we had watched and copied since we were old enough to walk and hold a baby doll. Or as we pretended to clean the floors and play shops.

We had been taught what it was to be someone who had a period and there was a stillness about finally arriving. What would this really be like?

Other girls I knew had already been bleeding for years before I first started. I would look at them and wonder what it was like to be them, to have a secret that people weren't supposed to find out. These girls seemed so other to me, so far beyond where I was. At least now I could join them in this secret club. I could flick my ponytail in a knowing way. I was one of them.

I had been given a brown paper bag with a pad in it when I was eleven years old, just in case. It was hidden down the bottom of my schoolbag and made me worried. We had heard about someone who had started to bleed on Year 6 camp. When we got home from the camp, all the girls were taken into a separate classroom and told that someone had started to bleed while we had been away. We shot looks around the room. 'Who was it?' we mouthed. We were told to be on the lookout for our own blood and that there were teachers who would support us if needed.

There seemed nothing more horrifying at that moment than the idea of being on the lookout for our own blood. Was it so unpredictable that it could arrive at any moment? I could sense how uncomfortable these conversations were making the adults around us. We had been spirited away to a private meeting that we knew should not be held in public.

This was what it felt like to keep a secret with each other. This first big secret is one of many that we learnt to keep. But it was shared with the other girls who sat there, trying not to give away how alarming it all sounded.

The suspicion that I and the other teenagers around me were regarded with confirmed that this was a danger we were entirely responsible for. We could ruin our lives and those of our families with what our bodies might do. We had to be careful now. The dangers were all around us. They whistled to us on the streets. They knew that we had this power, and they knew that it wouldn't take much if they felt like they might like to ruin everything – just a bit of fun, right?

Days and days were spent worried about what might happen if the blood were discovered. I can remember in high school when the oboe player stood up from her seat and we saw to our collective horror a bright, luminous red seeping through the back of her dress. I looked away. I couldn't bring myself to be the one to tell her and share in the horror of this exposure.

There were so many private rituals that took place in the smallness of my room. Hiding from the searing embarrassment at perhaps being laughed at for your attempts to feel comfortable with this changing self. Looking in the mirror at yourself from every angle. Could they see the pad? What if I bent down? There is sense of horror looking back at that time, filled with the utter vulnerability and self-hatred that comes with this sort of body secret. It wasn't just that you bled, it was that you were now a woman.

The hidden and private world of young girls is one that has long been fetishised. Even in the relative safety of our homes, young girls are sexualised.

* * *

In my forties when my periods first started to become erratic, an enormous grief rushed through me. The change that was beginning to take place inside me was unavoidably about coming to an ending of sorts.

What submerged me was how I had never accounted for this as something that I may feel as loss. It was like I had always understood that my menses was to be endured, a cross I needed to bear. But now there was a deep regret inside me that I had missed the chance to experience the potential and the beauty of that part of my life. I wasn't sure I was ready to leave the heartbreaking beauty of new life, the sense that you embodied something dangerous.

I felt that a large part of my life was over. And I had heard it was a torturous experience to go through both perimenopause and menopause proper. When I heard anything at all, that is. Like that of the very first period, most of the experience of menopause is shrouded in silence and secrecy. Right up until my mid-forties I didn't really know much about it. What happens? And how would it affect me?

All I had seen was some of my friends go through it. They were complaining of hot flushes that would keep them up at night and now sometimes found it difficult to complete work tasks. It seemed outrageous. Hadn't we been through enough? Hadn't our bodies dominated large parts of our lives both as objects and then in the ways they controlled our choices?

The life-giving force of menses and its conflation with the maiden that was leaving my body felt like a serious ending. I struggled to know what to tell my daughter about her own period because I had been so conflicted around the mythologising of this experience, this feeling that we were forced into claiming it as something to celebrate. With a group of my friends we took our daughters to a program developed to provide a safe environment for women and girls to talk about this time. I can't remember much except that I felt forced into presenting a softness – a wisdom, a beauty.

In reality, it should be about taking guns out into a field and shooting them into the sky. Covering our bodies in mud and howling at the moon. The time of life when you are cycling with the world is wild, it is connected, it flows with the universe in a way that is more powerful than we're ever taught to understand.

In this western reality, people who menstruate are taught to think of our periods as an extension of the way we understand ourselves as feminine: quiet, petite, small, defenceless. We are told the rage that fills us, like blood spilling into our mouths, is our darkness. This is the part that we must learn to push down and medicate. We feel so bad when it emerges in us because it has been pathologised. We've been told that it's not normal to feel like this.

My daughter and I shrugged at each other when we had finished the program. Were we supposed to make a banner when her period arrived so that she would feel proud? This was at such odds with a world that told her to hide it at all costs. Why are we expecting to have our daughters live in an alternate reality to the world that had already consumed them whole? How humiliating to pretend it was safe to raise banners and alert the world that her period had arrived. But where we live, the celebration is a forced denial of the reality that our girls who menstruate are entering a world of secrecy and shame. That they are in a world of inequity and danger.

And it's another time when we force an exclusion of our transgender women from an experience that is largely conflated with gender. Not all women menstruate; not all people who menstruate are women.

* * *

'Are you on your rags?' I heard a voice yell across the shopping mall. I spun around. Was he talking to me? I saw a group of teenagers sitting together laughing and looking at me. I was just entering the world that they were in. I was an awkward and clumsy teenager and was happy to go unnoticed. 'Are you a girl or boy?' he continued. I smiled widely, hoping this would disarm him, and gave them a thumbs-up. I had no idea what was going on. Was there blood on me somewhere? Could he see something? Why was he asking if I was a boy?

I kept going, pretending nothing he had yelled out had fazed me. But I knew my face would have turned bright red, and my heart was beating hard and had dropped deep into my stomach. I wanted to disappear. I figured he was just trying to humiliate me. And the ways he found that he could easily do it was to tell me I had a period and that I didn't even look like a girl should when I was having it.

He succeeded. I didn't want that sort of attention. I wanted to hide. Or to be one of the girls who was sitting with him, wearing their high-waisted jeans and laughing at me. They knew how to hide their rags and they knew how to look like a girl.

When my daughter finally got her period, she begged me not to tell anyone. 'I don't want to be the topic of conversation for the mums,' she said, sensing that there was a secret organisation of women sitting in the background taking notes and sharing experiences. She was right. We were always discussing the ways of our children, what had been good strategies, what we needed to avoid.

Older women often make the dangerous assumption that they share a sameness with the teenage girls in their lives. It becomes increasingly clear that any sameness is repulsive to those girls. We are too close. We can suffocate with the trying to know of the private worlds that they want to inhabit without the prying eyes of old women.

This is when the pushback begins. 'Don't think you know me' is the silent attack. 'Keep your distance or I'll scream' is the subtext. And we begin to sense that we don't belong together anymore. We are another type of woman, one that the teenage girls don't want to become. The sagging skin. The stomachs that roll over the top of our jeans, our loudness, our unawareness of just how disgusting we are.

Stay away, they mouth. Stay. Away.

* * *

No one had spoken to me about what would happen when my cycles would change and I would enter perimenopause. It was even more taboo than speaking about our blood every month. Menopause was a joke. The most humiliating time in a person's life, it would seem, when we should be avoided at all costs. And with these ideas firmly planted inside us, we approach menopause almost primed to play this role out.

Some women my age were describing themselves in the ways that I was feeling. 'Do you think it's perimenopause?' I would ask quietly. 'Dunno,' was often the answer. No one had any idea about what we should be looking out for, not really. And then, if we started to see the change, what should we do? That this was yet another change we needed to watch for around corners left us feeling like we were about to be under attack.

And while we were undergoing the enormous list of changes – thinning hair, drying skin, racing hearts, brain fog, sleepless nights, weight gain, panic, headaches, decreased libido, *to name just a few* – we were expected to keep a lid on it. Smile. Be amenable. Feel shame. Hide.

To be edging towards fifty and not have known about this change, to not really understand what we would be facing, seems absurd. To have it laughed about prepared us all for a state of being that we were afraid of. Embarrassed by. Satisfied to keep to ourselves.

My friend organised an online group for all of us around the same age, having realised that many of us were going through this at the same time. I was surprised that it hadn't occurred to me to do the same. But of course there were people I knew who would be approaching this same thing. Why hadn't I thought we should perhaps pool our talents and experiences and tell each other everything we knew and were learning, so we might find out a way to a collective understanding?

Horror stories were shared. I was introduced to the possibility of flooding, where blood will pour from you in such quantities that you might believe you were dying. There were stories shared of it happening to them, or their friends. One had taken themselves to hospital believing they were haemorrhaging.

It still felt as if we were sharing secrets, things we couldn't discuss with the wider world. Outside these groups we would continue to brush our hair, apply lipstick and head off to work, pushing down the growing rage. We would silently walk the house at night waiting for the hot flush to pass and say quiet prayers as our hearts skipped beats and felt as if we might be having a heart attack.

We sat together online and invited speakers to come to discuss the various ways we might approach menopause. There is always an undertone of politics with these decisions. Are you natural? Are you on HRT? Would you ever consider taking anti-depressants?

For women who go through menopause, it can feel like the transition from the wanted to the unwanted. What we had been convinced was the overt purpose for existence is clearly over. And it is in this vacuum that we are bombarded with ideas of what it means to age.

Darcey Steinke, writer and author of *Flash Count Diary: Menopause and the Vindication of Natural Life*, explained it beautifully in her article for *Time* magazine, 'I am a new creature, one closer to my former fierce little girl self. I feel a return to that essential me I had to leave behind once the huge disruptive force of puberty kicked in. I see now that my breeding years were an aberration rather than the norm. I can no longer reproduce but my body is far from over.'[1]

* * *

I went to visit a doctor to discuss the research I had done into the perimenopause symptoms I was having. Changed periods, carpal tunnel syndrome, increased asthma, sleeplessness, hot flushes, a sense that strong feelings would drown me, that I had lost touch with who I was and was afraid I would lose myself forever. He looked through me as I listed them off. 'I think I'll be the judge of what's going on with you,' was his basic response. 'Yeah,' I said, 'but this must have something to do with perimenopause, don't you think?' He smiled sympathetically. 'Well, we'll see.' I sat limply watching him ignore me.

I wanted to see if I could understand these changes in me differently. Not in an empty attempt to subvert them so that they no longer even resembled what they were, but to sit down deep inside them. What was this body memory that haunted me, this enormous grief and shame that washed over me every month and transformed into rage in an attempt to free itself from my skin, only to subside and lay quiet, ready to come alive again when the next month rolled around?

I was a slave to it for thirty-five years, sometimes riding the storm but mostly being drowned. That kind of cyclical grief is so difficult to understand. It is absent for large parts of the month and then embeds itself into the very centre of your life for a week, turning your world upside down, and leaves again. I never understood it. I didn't try to understand it. I was largely unconscious and would be dunked by its enormous wave each and every time it appeared.

We have been sold civility when this whole time we were meant to stay wild. Desiring to live deep inside the earth when we were given shoes to walk on top of it. We have been disconnected from the essence of our woman selves. We have brushed the wildness from our breasts and strapped them up so they won't bounce around. We have been broken like wild horses, trained and whipped to behave. Coaxed with treats if we do it the right way. Burnt at the stake if we do it the wrong way. Submit.

And here we were telling our young girls that they needed to behave, just the same way we had been told. To embrace the beauty of our changing bodies. But what about their darkness?

183

Why hadn't we been taught to embrace the dirt? The parts of us that were messy and didn't make sense? Instead, our periods were treated like gifts from fairies that were handed to us in little pink boxes.

What about images of blood-smeared thighs? And clots. And pain. And an aching that cuts through you like a knife, making you want to heave and throw up onto the wet earth. And cry. And heave and do it all again.

What were we so afraid of? That unkempt grief? The fear? The pain? If we didn't face it straight on, like I never had, it transformed into a blackness that wanted to feed on itself – it would turn on its host. 'Oh, it is you that is very ugly,' it would whisper into our bloodstream. 'You are lost. And dumb. And foul.' And that blood would pulse through our systems through the remaining weeks and get hot again when the month returned.

The silence that surrounds menopause is the same silence that surrounds all the secrets we keep. We hide ourselves down underneath the world so as not to rock the boat. To not frighten them with our power. To let them believe that they are not in danger from us.

But they are. Menopause has felt like the time when I should wake up from the stupid silence I had agreed to and realise that I had wasted all this precious time. All the time when I had been separated from my essential self. The time when I had been forced to forget where I really came from.

So perimenopause and menopause were at the heart of my ageing as I was forced to deal with the loss of my life as I had lived in the mother role. I hadn't permitted my own wildness that was still coursing through my veins. So I step into it now.

I grieved for what I had neglected in myself, the lost time of selfhood. But it also felt like a time of renewal. Of correction. Of allowance and acceptance of this wild state that I had been denied for so long.

Water

CHAPTER 12

Tsunami: Work

I OFTEN DREAM OF a tsunami. I see the waves gather on the horizon and I watch and wait for the wall of water to grow so high before it finally falls from the sky above me. It is always the same. I watch it build and build, knowing there is nothing I can do. It's too late now; there's no point in running or hiding. Very rarely do the dreams take me to my death, but I have died in them once or twice and travelled to a place beyond this one. It always feels the same when I wake up: the beauty and majesty of the ocean fills me in the same way as those dreams where I can fly.

* * *

When age has been strongly linked in our broader social lives to a loss of mental faculty, a heightened risk of health complications, an irrelevant perspective on social progress, a limited number of remaining years of service and a slower and less productive working output, older workers have a difficult time in proving their worth to prospective employers.

Some of the young people who start to populate your adult working life look through you. They know you don't understand the things they do, with access to the world at their fingertips. How could you? And they know they have the edge because they are prepared to risk it all for a better job. They haven't yet accrued the mortgage or the children or the reliance on a certain lifestyle or the understanding that you'll need to retire soon and you've got to make sure you will survive. So if they don't like something about the work they're doing, they'll say something or leave for something better.[1]

They haven't grown tired in quiet resentment like we have either, the fatigue of the relentlessness of work. The knowing that you are valued only while you are seen to be worthwhile. The endlessness of a working life. Decade after decade. Each day fuelled with a disquiet that you are not guaranteed this employment. That there is more to life than work. That there is a necessity to comply.

The landscape of employment opportunities has changed significantly for women over the past decades. Baby boomer women were not offered much scope in the employment available to them when they were young. My mum always said she could become a clerical worker, a teacher or a nurse – that was it.

I'm sitting with Fiona, a woman who's just clocked over into her sixties, who has just given me the painting that I commissioned of a dim sim being placed in my hands (it's a long story). As we talk, she remembers the overt barriers to the kind of work she really wanted to do when she was young. 'I wanted to be a sign writer but I was told that it was work only available to men. So I did the public service exam and became a draftsperson.' It took Fiona another thirty years to follow her heart and pursue her talent in art.

I study the painting that she's just handed me. 'It's so, so beautiful,' I tell her, knowing that she likely won't believe me. But it really is. She has captured a special moment for me and trusted in my absurd request. She underplays it. 'I'm just a housewife who paints,' she says, so impacted by years of feeling that she had no right to believe herself worthy of being told she is talented.

She worked only with men when she began in the public service. 'They would come and lean up into you, but you'd never talk about it. It wasn't something we thought we could mention. It was a different time.'

I ask her how she has found her experience of ageing, as I have asked most women I have encountered over the last couple of years. 'It's hard in this day and age. There is an inbuilt perception of what you should look like when you get old.' But now that she spends her days painting, she sees the world differently. 'When you paint, you need to see things as they really are. And there is so much beauty in the world when you look at it like this.'

The federal *Age Discrimination Act 2004* is designed to protect older workers, stating that no one should be 'discriminated against on the basis of age when advertising jobs; during recruitment and selection processes; when making decisions about training, transfer and promotion opportunities; and in the terms, conditions and termination of employment'.[2] But while there are legal protections within the Act, it is very difficult to prove age discrimination in the myriad of ways that it occurs in our workplaces. When our society and workplaces are so strongly focused on how we look, age becomes an enormous barrier. Due to the intersection of gender and age, the cohort most likely to bear the brunt of discrimination at work is women over the age of fifty.

Every single woman I speak to about writing on the experience of ageing points to themselves. 'Me,' they exclaim, 'talk to me,' wide-eyed and breathless with the revelations that ageing has brought. The treacherous path that it feels a woman over a certain age is expected to clamber, the danger that at any moment you'll be left without work or a family or safety or your home.

'Enjoy your next ten years of work,' Sally was told by a fifty-year-old co-worker. 'No one wants to employ an older makeup artist, not when you've got the pretty young ones to choose from. We're not good for business.' Sally was shocked when she first heard this. 'As if!' she says she thought to herself. 'Obviously that woman had other issues and was blaming it on age.'

But as Sally got older, she became more aware of the discrimination that she would eventually face. She saw it happening to women around her, and to protect herself she had decided early on to blame them. Were they too old and jaded now? Did they expect too much from their workplaces? As younger women made it into her industry, she saw that women who were seen as tired and old would be called last.

Then when Sally had a child she worried that the work wasn't going to allow her to be a mother, so she basically had to pretend she wasn't one and hadn't just given birth. Sally started making plans for what she needed to do going into the future. What would she have to learn to make sure that she and her son would survive once she hit fifty?

Emma Dawson, founder and Executive Director of the Per Capita think tank, has done the numbers. She cites research from the Australian Council of Social Service (ACOSS) and the University of New South Wales that in 2019 showed the majority of the world's poor are women, and Australia is no exception. Women face systemic barriers throughout their lives that make their poverty almost inevitable, and when we look at the lower-paid care industries that women are largely employed in – healthcare, childcare, aged care – we see the structural nature of gendered poverty. 'It is entrenched in our workplace settings and embedded in our personal relationships. It is at play at every stage of a woman's life, from childhood to the grave, making its mark on our education, our employment, our homes, our familial responsibilities and our retirement options.'[3]

The amount of time spent doing unpaid care work also links to the quality of the employment and the need to work in more vulnerable paid positions, such as part-time, casual and contract work. Dawson's research shows us that 'Most women earn less, are less likely to be promoted into senior roles, and more likely to take time off from the workforce and work part-time, to care for parents and other relatives than their male counterparts. In fact, Australia has one of the highest rates of part-time work for women in the OECD … For most Australian women, superannuation will not be sufficient for their retirement without the aged pension … Thirty per cent of single women over the age of 60 now live in income poverty, and that's directly linked to their retirement savings, or lack thereof. Unfortunately, there is now a rising trend of older women facing homelessness.'[4]

One of the most significant root causes of homelessness is poverty, and older women are more likely to find themselves in poverty due to systemic and structural discrimination in the workplace and cultural expectations that mean they are most likely to be the primary caregivers of children and older parents. 'There are few women who end their working lives having earned the same as, or more than, men working in similar employment.'[5]

The largest cohort of people in poverty around the world are women who also carry the largest burden of work in the caring industries. We see that care work is distributed unequally between women and men, with women providing the largest amount of unpaid care. Women are contributing almost double the amount of unpaid care work to that of men, and we see a direct relationship of this unpaid work to a lowered participation rate [of women] in the workforce.[6]

I had been trying to stay at university, but paying rent and bills was nearly impossible on the government student allowance. The only way that I could stick at it was if I also worked as many hours as I could. I was sick, though, and fatigued and starting to find it hard to keep up. When you're sick, the world doesn't stop for you, and social security benefits like the Disability pension are difficult to access. It took me a humiliatingly long time to wade through the bureaucracy and convince non-medical assessors that I needed assistance to survive. Even on the pension, I found it hard to pay my rent and bills. And when I had my first child, the cost of nappies and other items she needed meant we had to reconsider what was 'essential' each week.

The statistics are clear that women with disabilities are disadvantaged in their access to and maintenance of long-term, stable work. Very little has been done to ensure the equitable access to workplace opportunities for disabled people. It wasn't until the pandemic and the subsequent lockdown measures that led to big industries closing down virtually overnight, sending employees to work from home, that it became clear this degree of flexibility had always been possible. Flexible working conditions for illness, disability and caring had previously been hard won and was culturally frowned upon.

In Australia, single parents receiving a parenting payment are removed from that payment when their child turns eight. The theory is that children no longer need the level of parenting care they did, but parental advocates disagree. Analysis completed by the Parliamentary Budget Office has shown that no longer receiving the parenting payment support has saved the government over five billion dollars a year. It has meant that many single parents have been forced onto the lower Newstart payment. This has meant that the social cost of this 'saving' is women who were already living in poverty becoming even further marginalised with an increased inability to achieve a basic living standard.[7]

The impacts felt early on by women who spend productive periods of their lives as carers flows through the remainder of their lives. Having worked less while in part-time or full-time caring roles, women are in receipt of less superannuation. And while times are already tough for women who are single and surviving on reduced employment and benefits, the impact of this can be felt throughout the entirety of a woman's life.

When women disappear from the landscape as they age, the erasure is not only deeply insulting but utterly dangerous. If you can't see us, how do you know if we're lost? You can't see us if we're hiding to stay safe. Data from the Australian

Institute of Health and Welfare shows us that the fastest-growing group of homeless people in Australia is women over the age of forty-five. And the cohort most likely to miss out on homelessness support is women. It is an epidemic. What we also know is that these figures might not even be close to representing the actual number of women who are homeless, as those that are presenting at homelessness services are not often older women.[8]

After serving families as the primary caregiver, women enter older age with increased vulnerability. Traditionally, more women identify themselves as the primary carer and have less personal income saved and have accrued less superannuation. Often they are left vulnerable to marital breakdowns, death of partners or trauma and abuse.

Having had limited opportunity to build superannuation or purchase a home, getting older for an increasing number of women becomes life-threatening. But they are often unseen in the vastness of homelessness because visibility in this space for women can be dangerous. Often these women will find themselves sleeping in cars in suburban streets or carparks, or couch surfing if they are wary of homeless shelters for fear of abuse.

Further, women in this older age bracket are most likely to be the working poor, historically earning wages that were set to only three-quarters of their male counterparts. Writer and sociologist Ruth Quibell notes that 'For older women, poverty and housing insecurity is shaped by gendered social and economic inequalities which lay like traps, ready to make their full effects known in later life. Discrepancies in income with our male counterparts include a wage gap ... Lower pay rates in "feminised" industries show up over the course of a lifetime as lower earnings, savings and other forms of financial security.'[9]

Research shows that most older women who are homeless have never been homeless before. In fact, many don't self-identify as experiencing homelessness, viewing this as the stereotypical image of men sleeping rough.[10,11] And many women blame themselves for their homelessness. The blame lies squarely on a broken system.[12]

* * *

Founded in 1838, the Australian Club boasts members who are some of the most powerful politicians and business leaders.

While women are permitted entry as guests of male members, the club voted at a special general meeting in 2021 to 'consider a specific resolution for the purposes of amending the Club's Constitution to allow women to be Members', but the meeting 'determined that the 75 per cent threshold to pass the resolution was not met'. In fact, it was later reported that it had been a fairly resounding defeat of the proposition, where '693 member votes were cast, with 62 per cent against allowing women members, 37 per cent in favour and 1 per cent abstaining'.[13]

This is not, as some claimed, a quaint interest to have spaces that are safe for men, like a men's shed might enable, but absolutely about the denial of access to power for women. It's in these clubs that powerful relationships are formed and decisions are made about our civic lives. In 2021, the denial of women into this space is a clear indicator of the regard in which women are still held by some elites. That power rests in the hands of men, and while they may say all the right things in public forums, it is overwhelmingly in the interest of powerful white men for it to remain this way.

The other glaring omission from the Australian Club roll call is a cultural diversity of membership. One of the members of the club who remained anonymous when interviewed observed that 'You don't see a lot of Asian faces ... just look at the names of the members ... Howard, Hughes, Packer, Turnbull ... you don't see many Lis or Zhangs.'[14] This same exclusion is seen in boardrooms around this country where a minor reshuffle of the seats made available to women has been accompanied by only marginal changes when it comes to cultural diversity. A lateral power flow from white men to white women cannot be seen simply through the lens of gender equity as there is a significant intersection between power and whiteness.

White women have long had access to advantage and an adjacency to power via their relationship to white men. In Australia, colonial women were both colonised and colonisers. From the beginning of colonisation in this country, white women have not only taken advantage of white supremacy but also furthered its cause.[15]

When looking at the inequity in the workplace and the gendered access to power, it is essential to also acknowledge how our intersecting identities play a significant role in the level of discrimination we face. Race also plays a significant role in the experience of women in the workplace. To add insult to injury, there is a serious data gap in understanding the experiences of women of colour whose experiences are not specifically understood. But there is an urgent need for understanding the impacts of our identity intersections in our workplaces, as we know that women who identify from culturally and linguistically diverse backgrounds are over-represented in work that is both insecure and low paid. We also know that women who are migrants to this country are 7 per cent less likely to be employed than those born in Australia.[16]

And while we are all ageing within the paradigm of the patriarchy, we need to reconcile with the additional mechanisms of white supremacy if we are going to truly challenge its impacts. The consequences for women who are ageing is not equitable. Nor is access to power for all women on a par. We are separated into hierarchies of race, class, sex and gender identification.

Since colonisation, white women have not taken responsibility for their role in white supremacy, a bedfellow of patriarchy. White women have seen themselves as victims of the patriarchal project. But we must also account for how white women have served the advancement of the white patriarch. And by not challenging the unique intersections of race and gender identity, white women have been able to avoid the responsibility of their collusion to grab power and status alongside white men.[17]

White women function differently from men in the furtherment of white power, but they have played a significant role. As Aileen Moreton-Robinson describes in her seminal work *Talkin' Up to the White Woman*, 'white women civilised, while white men brutalised'.[18] Since the colonisation of Australia, white women have also been the beneficiaries of white supremacy.

And while white women have suffered at the hands of white men, they have played a pivotal role in ensuring the further subjugation of women of colour and First Nations women. They have been bystanders to the denial of access to the power domains that they themselves have accessed through this relationship to white male power.

While equity of access and discrimination in our workplaces is predominantly seen through a white lens, we are doing nothing to truly address the fundamental dangers for women as they age. It is one of our most urgent needs, to acknowledge and address women through an intersectional lens if we are to ensure that women not only have dignity as they age but that they are safe.

Water

CHAPTER 13

Abyssal Plain: Friendship, Love, Regret

THE LONELIEST WHALE IN the world lives in the North Pacific. It has been alone, as far as scientists have been aware since its call was first detected in the late 1980s. This whale calls at fifty-two hertz and is believed to be the only whale that emits a sound at this frequency. It swims back and forth across the ocean sending a signal out into a void, never having it answered. But it continues to call.

Every morning, for most of my life, I would wake up with a hum, a dark hum, that felt like there was danger somewhere. It was an ugly energy that swam deep inside the well of me.

* * *

I was discussing ageing on my radio show. The question I had asked is one that I was asking myself. Do you feel your age? What makes you feel old? What was clear from the responses we received was that many people felt that getting old happened in the body mostly, but not yet in the mind or in our imagination of ourselves. But that people, at some point, did begin to feel their age. There was a tipping point of sorts.

One woman rang in and did this thing that happens on radio: she sat with me and told me the truth. There is something about the power of this medium that makes it easier, I think, to tell the truth. No one can see you, but you know there are thousands of people listening and bearing witness. It's the perfect confession.

I can tell when a caller is going to do it. There is a calmness about them. A feeling that in a moment they might be unburdened by the thing that they need to say. For some of them, it seems to have been a long time coming. This woman was reflective and calm as she told me she was full of regret. It was that simple. There was no fighting this, or hoping it might be different, or even thinking she might do anything about it. Regret was knowing that you couldn't change your choices or an event, or a time in your life you wish had been different. Regret is that enormous pain of wishing it was different.

For her, it had been not heeding advice on some of the choices she had made when she was young. That she hadn't taken seriously health advice or listened when she heard her own body call to her to make a change. She was now living with cancer and, most likely, soon dying with cancer. But there was a tenderness in her regret. Somehow she had found space for that regret, as if she couldn't accept the life she had chosen but could accept the regret she now felt for it. She wasn't seeking to feel better or be absolved by sharing this, it was just a simple matter of fact: she wished she'd done it differently.

Hearing her speak like this knifed me. It felt an unbearable burden to imagine that we are living lives we might come to regret. That the choices we make may scar us – or, worse, others – forever. I think the pain of regret has to intersect with choice somehow. I'm not sure the pain of loss or of harm is the same pain that lives with you when that pain is known as regret. That it could have been different if you'd made a different choice.

'First, do no harm', the words uttered by some soon-to-be doctors. Not strictly from the Hippocratic Oath but embedded nonetheless into its folklore. There is a pervasive idea that on this earth we do everything we can to live well, and that alongside that we must also avoid harm of each other every step of the way.

We're encouraged to not have regrets. To live a life that has no evidence of this dark shadow lurking behind us. Why regret your life? Why harbour pain when it's avoidable? Ignore the storylines that continue to crop up in the middle of the night that cause you to sweat. Go harder. Do not listen to that voice that tells you you've done wrong. Keep moving forward. Do not look back.

I knew people like this who would look confused when I told them I felt badly about something. 'Why?' was often their response. 'They'll get over it.' They were right, of course, they would get over it. And I didn't have to understand the world the way I had been, full of me at the centre letting people down or embarrassing myself. Or just simply regretting the way I had gone about something.

The mantra encouraging us to live without regret is a strong one. Regret is treated as the anathema to living well. 'I don't believe in regrets' is almost the first answer to any question posed about the life we have undertaken. But bestselling author and former speech writer for Al Gore, Daniel H. Pink, believes there is something powerful about regret. 'Regret makes us human. Regret makes us better,' he argues in his book *The Power of Regret*. For the book, he undertook the world's largest regret survey with contributions by more than 15,000 people from around the world.[1] Pink argues that rather than denying it, regret can in fact guide us to live a better life. Processing difficult feelings like regret can assist us in learning more about who we are and what we really want in life.

But the experience of regret is painful. And as we age, the things we regret in our lives change somewhat. Our regrets become less goal-oriented and about missed opportunities and instead focus on health concerns or losing people we love. Crucially, one dominant regret in older cohorts is that of loss of friendships and the experience of loneliness.[2]

So aware was the UK government of the health impacts of loneliness on the older population that it was the first to install a Minister for loneliness.[3] One of the greatest impacts of ageing seems to be an increase in social isolation as a result of losing family and friends to death, deteriorating health that reduces mobility, increasing hearing loss and isolation from friends who may be challenged with similar experiences.

Such is the disregard for older people in our community that a royal commission was called to investigate the experience and safety of older Australians in aged care. The Royal Commission into Aged Care Quality and Safety (2021) found that at least one in three of those in residential aged care or using home care services had been subject to substandard care, including an incidence of assaults as high as 13 to 18 per cent. There is also a horrifying overuse of both physical and chemical restraint in residential aged care.

Throughout the royal commission the public was exposed to some of the treatment that had been going on behind the doors of residential facilities. The commission heard of 'physical and sexual abuse that occurred at the hands of staff members, and of situations in which residential aged care providers did not protect residents from abuse by other residents'. It went on: 'This is a disgrace and should be a source of national shame. Older people receiving aged care should be safe and free from abuse at all times.'[4]

The possibility that our lives might end in isolation, an aloneness that is imposed rather than sought, is suffocating. I find it hard to breathe at the idea that the life that swirls around me might one day be gone and I will be left alone. Similar to the process of understanding death, it is about understanding that everything here will one day be gone.

All the running around and busying ourselves and feeling as if there is no time in the day feels foolish in this light. At the end of all of that, there's nothing left but our breath and each other. There seems no grander objective, no greater success in our lives, than to have a hand to hold in those last years.

* * *

I was in a shower block in a caravan park last year listening in on two teenage girls who were sharing a shower cubicle. Their conversation was like two trees twisted together, so interwoven that you couldn't see where one began and the other ended.

They started and finished sentences as if their words shared an origin. It was as if they were, in fact, not two teenagers in a cubicle holding everyone up but one. 'Hurry up, girls,' yelled a waiting sunburnt woman impatiently. For a brief second they were silenced, and you could almost hear their eyes rolling and heads shaking as they whispered about the rude interruption.

Together, they had enough defence against the world to remain largely impervious. Together, they were mighty. They scurried out of the shower block, hair dripping, looking downward to avoid the eyes of the women lined up outside. When they got far enough down the dirt track that led to their caravan they began running and laughing.

* * *

I spoke to Susannah who told me about a friendship that had held her through an enormously difficult time. She met Hamish twenty-five years ago when she was at Melbourne University signing up for first-year sociology, that time in your life when the person sitting next to you during orientation week might end up being a person you know and love for the rest of your life.

Around seven years ago, Susannah's baby, Clementine, died, and Susannah's life turned upside down. At Clementine's funeral, dealing with his grief, Susannah's father filled the chapel with daffodils. And now, every single year around the time of Clementine's birthday, Hamish sends Susannah a photo of the first daffodil that he finds in bloom so she knows he remembers both Susannah and Clementine.

'Is it about bearing witness?' I asked Susannah. 'Yes,' she agreed. 'When you've lost someone, it's the friends who are willing to just sit with you. It takes such courage to witness and be with someone through that darkness and that mess. The people that are willing to step into that – who know that they are not going to fix it or that they're not going to make you happy, they're just going to sit here with you.'[5]

I spoke to Lesley, who wanted to share the story of a decades-long friendship. Her mother, now eighty-five years old and in a nursing home, lost her first child in 1962 to leukaemia. Since then, her mother's friend Margaret has rung her mother every single year on his anniversary. 'She doesn't always bring up why she's ringing, but she has never, ever forgotten. She still rings my mother now,' Lesley says.

Paula and Sandy have been best friends for over thirty years. 'What is it,' I ask as they sit easily with each other, 'that has meant that you've been able to keep this friendship through the enormity of life and all its changes?' Without much hesitation, they both agreed that it's a shared history. Not having to explain to each other the life that has built each of them. The small moments and the big moments that make up the whole.

Are the states of regret and loneliness and friendship all wound together somehow? Our loneliness can be reframed, and with its prevalence perhaps we have no option but to ensure that we find a way to see the experience differently. But the most heartbreaking aspect of ageing for me is that we might end up alone and lonely.

ELEMENT:

Earth

Endings

Earth

Introduction

GRAVITY HOLDS US ALL earthbound. I am held here too, not against my will exactly, because I can't remember it being any other way, but there is something inside me that yearns to lift off the ground. Like so many, I am left only with dreams that I can fly.

It's always the same dream: I pump my arms hard so I'm using every muscle, as if I might be strong enough to do it, to really do it – to lift off the ground. And sure enough, slowly I gain enough momentum and am rushed with the familiar feeling that it brings me every time I fly: freedom. I can go as high as I desire, and when I wake, I have the sky in my heart and feel as though I might really be magic.

I have seen the world below from that tiny window in a plane as it might be seen by a bird. In those moments I try to block out other people and pretend I am alone in the sky. And when we eventually fly over my city from such a great height it is a glistening sea of lights, a mass of indistinguishable beauty.

From up here it looks like how it feels to love this place. Then we drop from the sky just enough to etch out the mundanity of houses and cars and roads and I feel the heartbreak of landing, when you realise you are back on earth and you can only see the world from where you stand. The rotten trick of being earthbound is that when I'm on the ground again, it doesn't take long for the smallness of me to be forgotten. I forget that I'm just a tiny part of the huge world that I saw from the sky. It doesn't take long to forget the enormity of it all and to believe that maybe the entirety of the world is only what I can see, and that I'm a much bigger part of it all than what I really am.

* * *

Before the Ash Wednesday bushfires in 1983, the earth along the eastern and south-eastern parts of Australia was dry. When we dug down, the soil crumbled between our fingers like powder. When the earth is this dry it pulls away from itself. I felt like if I wasn't careful, I might fall between the aching cracks and be swallowed whole.

This drought, which started five years earlier, was at its most intense in the year before the fires came through. Unlike other natural disasters, a drought happens silently and slowly. It is the natural disaster that affects most people globally but attracts the least amount of alarm from those not directly impacted. No TV ratings are won without raging fires, or rumbling earth, or wild wind. A drought is just the quiet, slow, insistent denial of all life.

Drought is an absence. It is a heart that is waiting, waiting for the blood that may never arrive. Some droughts that have dried the earth skin of this country have gone on so long that teenagers have rarely seen or felt the rain. They don't know about the relief that the rain will bring not only to the earth but to the wildness that lives inside them.

* * *

When I was eight, I would spend hours digging in my front yard, trying to find where everything began, half wondering if it might really be possible for me to dig through to the other side of the world. My fingers would sting as I scratched against the hard ground. I could feel the burn of the cold air that had seeped into the ground.

In that same dirt lived creatures that I didn't want to touch. A boy once chased me around the schoolyard with a worm, threatening to throw it on me. I felt terror. Not confected terror that you would sometimes amplify to encourage the drama but real body-shaking terror that he would catch me and put the worm down my dress. It was a horrible idea, a wet worm covered in the earth that it had been plucked from.

My brother showed me how worms could be cut in half and create two new worms. As he sliced them with a shovel, I imagined what it might feel like to have a spade descend from the heavens and cut you in two. Perhaps it is the reverse of what we're told a human yearns for, that we begin as a half until we find the other part that will make us whole.

Later on I learnt that when earthworms are cut in half they don't really live to become two worms. Instead, the head might survive and grow another tail. But more likely it will die. I also learnt that a human doesn't need another half to become a whole – we are born complete.

In that same front yard, I fell in love with a tree. It was the only tree that grew tall on our small neighbourhood block, a lonely tree in the suburbs that helped me remember I wasn't the little house where I lived. Or all the problems I was having at school. The tree was a reminder that a kid doesn't need much to take them back home to the stories of the wind or into the earth. It doesn't take much to light our remembrance of where we began and where we belong.

Within this tree's canopy lived my everything as I played and climbed and imagined myself into life. Its limbs kept my secrets, ones that I barely noticed I was whispering to myself. I was sure I could feel that tree, as if it could be known to me. That it was kind. That it was my friend. That it, in turn, also liked me. And as the light lowered over middle Australia, I spent hours and hours inside it, becoming who I am.

In the autumn its leaves would transform from green to a brilliant gold, and then, in a final performance, my tree would end it all by dropping every last one. The leaves would be thick on the ground, and I would spend hours raking them up into an enormous pile. I would roll around inside them, covering my body in its wet, slimy remains.

I read about this tree and its kin like you might learn about any ancient culture. Golden ash. *Fraxinus excelsior* 'Aurea'. Drought-resistant so less concerned that the earth was drying. It had learnt to survive and had not much sympathy for the trees that didn't know how. In winter the branches birthed black buds, and while dreaming for hours I would pull them off and scissor them apart with my sharp fingernails.

My tree came from a noble clan. In Norse mythology, Yggdrasil was a sacred ash tree said to support the entire universe. Its branches extended to the heavens and its roots extended across the entirety of the worlds: the underworld, the land of giants and the home of the gods. From root to leaf, the ash stretched from the depths of hell to the gates of heaven.

The ash is also found in Celtic mythology, where it is thought to connect the inner self to the outer world. Similar to Norse mythology, the Celts knew the ash as the world tree, connecting above and below, and as one of the five sacred trees that stood guard over Ireland. When babies were born they were 'sometimes given a spoonful of Ash sap' because it was believed to 'prevent disease and infant mortality'.[1]

My tree was there the day I left that house when I was seventeen years old. For as long as I lived there, its cycles stayed the same. It didn't alter its course or change in any considerable way. At least, not a change that I understood or had noticed. Year in, year out, it was heavy in the earth. And like that tree, I felt like I was the same girl whenever I was with it.

After raking up the leaves each autumn with my brothers and sister, my dad would throw them in the incinerator out the back and I would watch the black smoke dance into the sky. This was one of the tree's many deaths. And for those months my tree sat quiet, silent almost, like it had nothing to do but wait to be reborn.

* * *

When I think about how we age and die and are returned to the earth, I think of that word 'returned'. How are we returning to this elemental force? Returned to the site of bounty and of nurture, to be dead inside the world. How does the world encounter our death like this? Tucked inside itself, our rotting corpses leech their remaining life force into the soil.

Eventually you learn that everything is connected. In fact, the real lesson is that there is no separation. When the rain soaks my hair or I push my finger into the wet dirt and feel like I am inside it, I whisper to remind myself, 'I am that too'.

Now that I had been picked up and landed in an older version of me, I wondered what I should do with the chaos that I had found myself in. I was beginning to look back through the wreckage and wonder about dealing with regrets about the life that I had lived. Regrets that woke me up in the middle of the night during that hour when witches roam the skies, making mischief and terror. Regret for all the things I was too frightened to do. Or too slow. Or too self-critical. Or when I went too hard and didn't wait for others to catch up, or made a mistake in what I thought was important, or listened to the wrong people. Backed the wrong horse.

It is in the earth that I discovered that when we age, the world can turn us upside down. We need to reconcile with the pain we have caused and the pain that has been inflicted upon us. This is the final shedding, the final storm before we can make our way to the end.

This is the silence and the reflection on our death as we quietly wait to be reborn.

Earth

CHAPTER 14

Buried: Mind

I KNEW I WAS going to age, but I didn't really understand how it would be possible when living seemed like such a static state. All the old people I knew had always been old, and for a long time. I would see those wrinkly faces as belonging to people who were not me. It was impossible to imagine they were faces that could have once been like mine. They were old and I was young. We were, without question, distinct types of people.

'Poor old people,' I thought, and pledged to think of them kindly if I ran into them on the street. I would look like I was listening and was interested in their stories of the 'olden days' when they wore second-hand clothes and rode ponies to school. I thought of old people as an oddity. They had gone to the war, or had survived a pandemic, or had lived in other countries and had escaped from violence to live here. These were stories that belonged to other people and had nothing much to do with me at all.

In my Year 9 class we'd been encouraged to visit an old people's home – that's what we called it, a home where old people lived. A distant land that was hidden from view, out of sight, out of mind.

We were encouraged to go there as an act of charity, as if our attendance at the home would be a noble sacrifice of sorts. Visiting old people was what a good, kind citizen would do, like picking up litter or making sure you paid your parking ticket on time. It was never framed as anything that might, in fact, be a reciprocal affair. We were never expected to think that perhaps we might gain something from being with humans who were older than us.

My nana Lesley ended up in a home like this when her dementia finally became too difficult to be managed at home. Visiting her, I would walk through the doors and be arrested by the smell of urine hidden in the walls and the floors. The smell took on a life of its own after being doused with disinfectant and various odour busters to try to arrest it. But it was there, like a cancer in the carpet and the curtains.

It was confronting to see 'old people' everywhere, shuffling down hallways and semi-reclined on big chairs in common rooms. We had done such a good job of hiding them from our regular lives in these types of places that you could almost be forgiven to think that old people, like these, didn't exist. The smells frightened me. The decay frightened me. The absence of my real nana frightened me. This woman who was standing in for her still carried my nana's love, but I didn't know then how to navigate such a changed person. I didn't know how to let go of who I was, to allow her to become this fluid and everchanging version of herself.

Spending time with her, seeing how she lived, how everyone lived around her, made it very clear that we became elderly and not elders in the white culture I was living in. Friends who came from other cultures treated the elders in their families differently. First Nations friends, for instance, would fill me with shame that I did not regard my elders as they did. Regardless of familial connection, there was clearly a belief that all elders deserved respect from them.

Lois, a Yorta Yorta woman, describes it for me: 'In the Aboriginal community we have this thing about respect for Elders, and acknowledging their journey and their wisdom and their cultural knowledge and so forth. And so there's an expectation that younger people acknowledge that, and that's how the "aunty" comes into it. It comes from the community who just suddenly start to call people aunty or uncle, whatever the case may be, because they recognise and acknowledge what people have done, you know, in their private journey. I'm privileged to say that I do hold knowledge from through my family line, as an Aboriginal person, that has kept me in good stead of who I am, how I should do things, you know, the cultural framework and how I work, the values that have been handed down to me about the importance of relationship, responsibility and respect. And those things I hold very dear to me.'[1]

* * *

When I was growing up, my nana Les would sit in a big beige lounge chair in front of the heater and spend hours thinking about words while she did the crossword. She was beautiful and gentle and dignified. She had the most incredible head of hair and the softest skin that barely wrinkled. But she always seemed old to me. And I think she saw herself that way too.

When she became a grandmother, I guess she understood that grandmothers looked a certain way. The times were slowly shifting to a more modern interpretation of what being old might look like, but it was almost a cultural and social contract that you must look the part. There would be bags and gloves and coats and hats for special occasions and games of bridge in the front room, the good room, with the ladies from church.

She wasn't alone – I think a lot of women in her generation were convinced that the world should work like this. Oldness was inevitable and fitted into the life span they were expecting. It was a pathway that made sense from the many years they had spent rearing children and keeping houses. There was a certain appeal to how simple this made things: clear, distinct roles for the living of their lives. She can't have been that old, though, thinking back and doing the maths. She was less than seventy when she was dressed up in her old lady clothes.

When I was little, we would catch the number 6 tram, a rattler, from outside the front of her house. We would sit neatly on the wooden slats of the bench seats, as we headed to the city, where there was always a buzz of excitement. She would take me out for lunch and buy me a new outfit, and I would spend most of my time just watching her. It seemed to me that the world belonged to her, that she knew her rightful place and was comfortable there. She held herself strong and I felt safe trailing behind her. Going into the city like this was a job that needed to be done together.

There was the smell of the supermarket when we would go shopping together for her weekly groceries. I can see the sparkly floor and the excitement of maybe getting a treat, a small packet of chips or a fizzy drink. And every Sunday night my family would gather around her table and have a meal together. We did this for decades.

And then, without much warning, dementia took hold of her mind and her body. The woman I had spent my life watching and loving was suddenly gone. I was older by then and understood that this could happen to people when they aged, but I didn't account for the confusion of losing someone who was still there in front of me.

I would look for her in every movement. I would stare into her eyes and hope to see even a flicker of her old self, just enough to know that she had become lost somehow, and if we all tried hard enough, we'd find her again and she could come home.

She would appear sometimes and I would be flooded with an urgency to tell her to stay. To tell her everything that had been happening while she had been gone. But as soon as she returned, she would be gone again without warning. And then, like every time before, she would be lost somewhere else where the storyline of her life was entirely different from what we knew it to be. Her eyes would cloud over and she would leave me.

We were still in her story but just played a range of different characters. Sometimes my mother would be her sister; sometimes my dad would be her husband. One thing she always had a sense of was that we played characters in her life who loved her, we were just mixed up.

It didn't happen overnight. When she first started showing signs of this mental decay she would panic. Why couldn't she remember the name of that thing? Why had she forgotten her reason for travelling to the shops down the road? She knew what happened to some people when they got old and could sense there was a change up ahead, and she was frightened of it. She knew this would mean suffering a kind of death before her body had decided it was her time to die.

Losing her like this catapulted me into questions about everything. Who was this Lesley I thought I knew? She still smelt the same, and her smile was less sure, but it was still hers. Her voice was still soft, and her laugh came from her heart, like it always had. But she didn't share the same version of the world with us anymore. 'Did that matter?' I wondered. 'Did it make her less her?'

The myth that the cells in our body die and are renewed every seven years has led many to wonder how, if we are changed like this at a cellular level, we can claim to be the same people we were seven years before. The truth is a little less neat. Our body has somewhere between fifty and seventy-five trillion cells that actually renew at different rates throughout our lives, but perhaps the question of selfhood is still relevant. If we are changed at a cellular level from the day we are born, what can we claim to be the self? Who is this 'me' I refer to? And if it's not our matter or our minds, what is it?

As we get older and the outer shell becomes unrecognisable from the body that ran around at seven years of age, how can we claim to be the same person? Does this physical change render us different? Or does our body have much less to do with the self than we give it credit for?

The other day my son asked me a classic philosophical question: if the truck you have been driving has needed every single part of it replaced over time, is it the same truck? Like the continuous self, if we are constantly renewing, then is the body that I had as a child different from the one I'm walking around in now? Am I the same truck?

So I returned to this idea of our memories. How important are they, as we age, to the sense that we have had a continuous life? A life that can be linked and evolved and developed from the moments that have come before? I wondered if it's not memories that connect our various selves over time but the *feeling* of what it has been to live in this body, feelings lodged inside us that don't belong to words or a story anymore. They are just what it *feels* like to be us.

I have also wondered if it is our pain that makes our selves feel continuous. There is pain inside me that I have carried for decades, mostly it is unseen but sometimes you can see it on my body: a scar, a sallow cheek, eyes that sit low and sad on cheekbones. I think as much as we believe that we want to be rid of our pain, that we wish to relinquish ourselves of it, I think that pain is something we can find difficult to release. How would it feel to be ourselves without it? The pain comes to feel as much you as anything else you harbour in your body.

Are we the person that is carried through all the changes that happen to our bodies and our minds as we age, the one that remembers how to feel the pain?

When I look in the mirror, I feel like the girl who once lived on the outside of me, all alive skin and shiny lips. I can feel how it hurt to be her, and this particular pain is shared with others that know themselves this way, the same way we know what it feels like to be expected to walk in high heels – the absurdity of this torture as our feet are squeezed into an impossible shape and asked to balance on a thin platform.

What else have you got?

We are more likely to carry pain through our lives than memories of simple joy or happiness. Intergenerational trauma is finally being understood as it pertains to trauma inflicted on whole communities and how that is passed through our very blood. So encoded is this trauma, now alive in a new body, it can be difficult to know how to understand that pain as you. It is transferred through violence, through continued trauma, through the sharing of unimaginable pain.

Is this what connects us to the selves we thought we had left in the past, the little children we once were, the teenagers we thought we'd always be? They live with us. They always feel like they are us. And I don't want to leave them back there, I want them to come with me. I want to know myself as continuous. That while I age and decay there is a thin wire that joins all these bodies together, that makes me whole.

And while the pain dominates my body memory, maybe it is also feasible to imagine that it could be the joy that winds our separate selves together. The birthday candles we blew out. The holidays at the beach where we got lost in the enormity of building a sandcastle. The first crickets coming out on a summer's night. The different shapes of the moon that you begin to understand as a cycle.

We spend an enormous amount of time both in our memories of ourselves and in the imagination of what we might become. We travel back to vast horizons of our lives using a faulty cognitive system called a memory to construct who we were and then who we believe ourselves to be now. The understanding of what we were constructs the idea of who we believe we are; adjust those memories and you have a different self. Changing the story you believe about your past can drastically impact your future.

The ancient Greek philosopher Aristotle argued that our ability to conceive of a past is vital to the understanding and imagination of our future. The ability to move backwards and forwards is how we can create new ideas. Every idea connects in some way to the past. Nothing is new. It has emerged from somewhere.

So I kept circling back to Lesley. If we erased our memories, as my nana's had been, how would we understand the world around us and our relative place within it? Is there something that is vitally who we are that exists beyond memories of self? Can we construct the world and our lives within it, the way we might like them to be? A false life? A better life? Who would argue? All the regrets that have wedged themselves into your heart, a tiny knife each of them, might be easily removed. Our memories charge our bodies with the enormous emotions that fill us. They wake us up at night and have us sweating with regret. Why did we make that decision? Or why did we fail to decide?

There was a wonderful story about a woman who suffered brain injury and memory loss who fell in love with the same man she had been married to years before. Not remembering anything of their life together before her accident, she found herself falling in love with the same man.[2] What does this tell us about the intrinsic self? That there is one? But how much clarity do we need to find it? How do we ignore the stimulus from the outside to connect with the real us on the inside?

What is it about that little girl that feels exactly the same today as I look at how her body has changed? She is the same inside me, though long gone. Would anyone recognise her who once knew her? Does it matter?

* * *

I had spoken to Lena about her family at various times since we met, and in those conversations she would often describe their dynamic as 'complex'. Lena lives in a different city from her family now, far enough that she could forge her own story and make her own family. She was the youngest of seven and her mother, the matriarch of the family, had always been elusive to her.

'For my whole life, we've never really spoken. She doesn't speak English and I can't speak Arabic enough to have a proper conversation with her. Since I was five years old, my brothers or my sisters would have to translate for me. I can understand her but she can't understand me, and I've never been able to express myself to her – she's never known who I am. We've never had a real conversation with each other.'

The language barrier had created an enormous space between them that has continued through the entirety of Lena's life. But recently, Lena visited her mother for the first time in a number of years after learning that her health had deteriorated and she was developing dementia. 'I was sitting there with her, and I realised after she asked me a few questions that she just didn't know who I was. She knew I was Lena, but she didn't remember our life together.' For the first time in her life, a weight lifted off her. 'Afterwards I cried and cried. It just felt like everything could be let go of. If she didn't remember everything that had been lost between us, why was I carrying it?'

Months passed between that first meeting and a call from Lena's brother to tell her that her mother was in ICU, Lena raced to be by her side, 'There's been two times in my life where I've been mute. The first time was the death of a small baby and the second time was sitting with my mother in her hospital bed. I couldn't say anything, so I sat with her in silence. Just like we had our whole lives.'

* * *

My nana remembered songs we had sung with her as children. 'She's a pretty little dear, she lives uptown, her daddy is a butcher and his name is Brown. Her beauty is of high renown, she's the girl for me.' It was an old song the children in our family are taught almost as soon as they are born. Somehow it stayed with her, deep down inside the woman who had loved us all when she sang it with us. In that place we can all feel what it is to be connected to each other.

I transcribed one of our conversations, which I had recorded for a philosophy class I was taking at university. Her voice is held in time on this recording, and it feels like I still have her somewhere. This woman who had changed in so many ways still has the voice of the woman we grew up with. That was the difficulty: she still sounded and looked the same, but the woman inside had different memories from the ones we might have shared with her. She had a different sense of the boundaries of life, and in some ways this new version of her was much freer, entirely less self-conscious.

What would have happened if I had been able to go down further than our shared experience of memories, down to the place where we exist beyond time and space, to the place we connect to each other? I guess that's what music is for, a feeling or an energy we can share that doesn't mean we need to share a history.

In this one recording we talked for hours, and in detail, about her life as a race car driver. About how she had worked hard, how she had been well regarded, how she had had to watch her rivals because they were always there, ready to take her spot at the top of the table. That day was the only time I heard this story and it was watertight. She knew it inside and out.

I began to wonder if there was some truth in what she had been telling me. Had she really had a life as a race car driver? Was it possible that we didn't know everything about her? Before her children were born, the ones who had been keeping her history alive, had she lived a life that no one knew about?

It seems absurd now to have wondered. We knew she had worked at the Australian Mint before she met her husband, but it brings up the question of our memories and how we use them to understand our present. If you remember your life as a race car driver, if you believe this with your matter and your skin, is this the life you had? Where else does the truth of our lives exist if not in the feelings those memories give us? Are we more than the memories we've constructed about our lives? Does it matter if those memories are accurate?

Science has long shown us that our memories are likely to have elements of construction. The way we embed memories relies upon how we need to make sense of them. The American psychologist Elizabeth Loftus changed the way we understand this by theorising that our memories were not being replayed *to* us but rather constantly being reconstructed *by* us. 'It is not fixed and immutable, not a place way back there that is preserved in stone, but a living thing that changes shape, expands shrinks and expands again, an amoeba-like creature with powers to make us laugh, and cry, and clench our fists. Enormous powers – powers even to make us believe in something that never happened.'[3]

Recently, Loftus controversially testified for the defence in the trial of convicted sex offender Harvey Weinstein with theories that may have lead the jury to believe that some of the women testifying may have recast neutral or disappointing sexual encounters with Weinstein as abusive after revelations had emerged publicly about his predatory history.

Obviously problematic for many of us that this sort of research can call into question everything we believe happened in our lives, because it becomes difficult to recount any experience as true. If this is the case, how is it possible to have no reference that can travel back, nothing that we can trust?[4]

So how do we understand this in our own contexts? How different are the lives we have lived from the ones that we remember? And if we remember something different, something that helps us live a better life now, is that okay? If all our memories are partially false, perhaps we should use that to our advantage. Or, better still, leave the idea of memories behind. Understand that there is nothing back there that we need to bring into our present. Make the story new every day.

Earth

CHAPTER 15

Kairos: Time

TIME IS ONE OF the great enemies of our life force, though it is sometimes difficult to think of it this way. I have spent a large portion of my life wishing that days would run faster. Or that a job that I had undertaken would be over so I might go to bed. Or that I could sleep through pain and sickness. I had been willing my life to be over faster in all those micro moments where living seemed mundane or too hard to endure, allowing days to roll into each other where one becomes difficult to distinguish from the next. I have been slow to understand how to cherish every day.

The ancient Greeks had two words for time, *chronos* (χρόνος) and *kairos* (καιρός). *Chronos* refers to chronological or sequential time, while *kairos* is said to signify an opportune time to take action. *Chronos* is quantitative; *kairos* has a qualitative, permanent nature and sets itself apart with a belief that there is

226

something as magical as 'right timing'. We live through hours and minutes. But we *live* and we are alive if we understand the concept of *moments* and that there is more to time than a unit of measure.

Moments feel like they might still be alive inside us. The moments that don't age – the moments we can return to as if they happened yesterday – belong in our bodies, and we can find them if we search hard enough. We can embody those moments and imagine we are still there. The moment I hid inside the clothing rack at a department store and let my mum think she had lost me. The moment I drove the car to hospital through silent streets at 5.30 a.m., on the way to give birth to my second child. The moment I ate a hot chilli for the first time and my whole system felt like it was in collapse.

In contrast, perceiving our lives in hours and minutes is what takes those magical *kairos* moments and transforms them into the march of time, the unrelenting crawl forward. *Chronos* removes the ephemeral dimension of time, reducing our experience of it by doing something we perhaps should never have done – count it.

I can hear the ticking of the clock that sat on the ornate mantelpiece in my grandparents' home, the bell chiming at the top of the hour to remind me exactly where I was in the day. It's lunchtime. It's almost bedtime. The warm, reassuring sound, the cooing 'dong' that wouldn't allow me to forget I was a human that was both vertical and horizontal. With a clock I can only move forward or backward in time. Any sense that I could drift off in my imagination into a vertical world is quickly deadened when I know the time. I am quickly arrested back into the sense that time has captured me.

Some have argued the clock is the most significant machine used during the industrial age. It improved our seafaring navigation with the development of the marine chronometer and enabled the invention of GPS and mobile technologies. But our reference to clocks and calendars changed the way we observe matter in relation to time. How old we are is told to us by a system of time that ticks over every single day, twenty-four hours at a time, 86,400 seconds a day.

I did the maths on my own life. It has been 17,063 days since I was born. I have slept a total of fifteen years of that time. I have been alive for 409,512 hours and 24,570,720 minutes.

When I was born, nurses told my mum that my cries sounded like that of a duck. It's a story I've heard dozens of times through my life.

My own children have asked me to tell them about their births. I have found it harder to share the details as they are still shrouded in the trauma of that closeness I felt we had all come to dying. But the way we enter the world is significant. We count every year from that date. Our birthday, the day we were born, is celebrated by everyone who loves us. Every year we acknowledge how much joy it brings to have people born into our lives.

And every year, on that day of birth, we count how many years we've been here. To begin with, we are desperate to be older, impatient to bypass the particular limitations that being a child brings. At first it's the excitement of getting to double figures. And then it's the desperation to be considered a teenager.

And then we cannot wait to be considered an adult, away from those foolish teen years when we had haircuts and wild ideas that embarrass us now. And soon enough comes a point where we wish that the birthdays would stop and we could be considered young again. We whisper our age when someone dares to asks, because it is considered rude to enquire. Your best bet, if you're ever asked how old you think someone is, is to take ten years off what you really think.

But what if we were never told about age in that way? How would we relate to the feeling of being a human in the moments that we have?

We learn to ask 'when will we get there?' almost as soon as we can speak. I know that I am often thinking about being anywhere but here in this moment. And the older we get, the faster every moment seems to travel by. 'Where does the time go?' I wonder, and then realise I have been doing everything to will it all away, to get to the next bit, the next day, the next moment.

How old do you feel? It is a question that is supposed to illuminate more about your health and wellbeing than knowing your calendar age. When you close your eyes and dive down into how it feels to live in your body, what is it like? How old does it feel to be you? Can you tell the difference between the you that lived twenty years ago and the you that lives now?

Of course, the answer will depend on the day and your physical state at the time, but research has shown that many people feel much younger than their chronological age, often up to twenty years younger. What was also interesting about these studies was that even if the participants advised they had at least one chronic illness that impaired the quality of their lives, they were still capable of experiencing age as younger than their chronology would explain.[1] Which is interesting when we consider how much older chronic illness can make us feel.

* * *

Einstein's discoveries changed everything people thought they knew about time. Rather than believing that time flowed in one direction, he understood that time was relative, so that depending on your frame of reference, time passes at different rates. Some scientists have taken this idea further to propose that time is an illusion. But the power of our perception of time remains.

What does this say about how we anticipate age? What is the feeling of age? Is feeling young the buzz in your stomach on Christmas Eve when you were seven years old? Is feeling young about finding access to wonder and awe? To be overwhelmed by something beautiful or profound that takes your breath away? Discovery? Love?

Is getting old when the world doesn't seem new anymore? Or when the physical decay of your body and mind means you change the way you interact with the world? Or your physicality changes the way you think of yourself? This is the end, they tell you. Suck it up.

When we look into the world and feel as if we have already seen everything there is to see. When we stop looking deeply to find joy. When we stop seeking to hear new music. Or to find a new outfit to wear. Or to draw pictures. Or play in the dirt. We stop because we don't think these activities belong to us anymore.

That daydream that I would always have of me, the person who lived inside my imagination, filled me up so that I was entirely her. I was avoiding looking at the face that didn't match how my insides felt. It has always been a shock to see photos of myself. Shocking and disappointing. The image that

I walk around with is blurry and more a composite of how it feels to live in this world. I have developed a strong self-esteem based mostly on how I imagine I am.

Philosophers have long wondered about the nature of the self. Who are we? Are we the same person as the child that suckled on a chest? A small child that undertook a dense series of codifications to know herself as a girl, the hair, the dress, the lips, the attraction to colour? Are we the teenager that rebelled and believed the world was a wicked place determined to dampen the spirit? Or are we the inevitability of our future selves? Or the person we are consciously moving forward to become?

Ageing is the experience of matter moving through time. We have been taught that life is a journey, and we are the travellers on a long, straight road. As we get older, we realise there is more behind us than ahead of us. When we know ourselves to be more past than future, who are we that stands at the crossroads of that timeline?

The body is a finite organism. It has a beginning, and it has an end.

* * *

I somehow already knew about living and dying in my body. It must be programmed in us before we arrive on earth. I drove onto a block of land that my friend owned in the Grampians, on Gunditjmara country. It had taken us about four hours to get there, the final part of the trip down a long and bumpy dirt road that I navigated as best as I could in my beaten-up European car. I was dripping in the detritus of a city life, my head full of conversations and ideas and meaningless songs that took turns to hold my attention. Endless thoughts that removed me from where I was and what I was actually doing. I was living in my mind.

It was nothing remarkable; in fact, it was how I had always lived, with my head and my heart far away from where I was. Sometimes dropping back in to see what was around me but always with a sense of someone watching in, not living here.

I drove the car up the steep driveway to the shack, reminding myself to breathe in the air but already planning when I would leave in a couple of days. Not because I didn't want to be there but because I was always working multiple steps ahead, thinking I knew how the world would twist and turn and how I would navigate it. Endless lists. Endless ideas that rumbled and rattled around in my head. Never a moment of silence.

But it was almost immediate. When I opened the car door and stepped out onto the earth, I had an overwhelming sensation of belonging. It is something we have heard spoken of by the First People, who have lived close to the earth for thousands of years, but it was new for me. It was a feeling that made so much sense but didn't have a language I had ever known. How to explain that deep knowing inside your body? Beyond thought. Beyond ideas. Beyond the rumble of my mind. Beyond time. I knew something about where I was that I couldn't describe.

There was a feeling inside my body that all the things outside were also inside. That it was all suddenly clear. The city didn't make sense to me here, the concerns that I had there. The stress. The obsession with small things and with my screen. In one sudden swoop I had been transformed. And I remained that way until I left a few days later.

Is time the element we need to combat if we hope to be free of our ageing? Do we need to spend more of our lives not looking, not counting, not assessing ourselves against the concepts that time imposes on our lives?

Illness arrives and reminds you that you've been living the lie that your body would just persist. That it would just continue to be like this, always. We can barely look upon the decomposed human form; it is the stuff of nightmares and horror films. The notion that our bodies will be burnt to ashes or lie in six feet of cold earth to slowly be eaten by bacteria and bugs is a violence we refuse to face.

When we are finally forced to understand that our bodies will break, we can no longer hide from the truth-telling of our own mortality. What seems so horrifying is nothing but a beautiful twist, but at this point it is impossible to see it that way.

Earth

CHAPTER 16

Autolysis: Returning

MY GRANDFATHER'S CASKET SWUNG ever so slightly as it was being lowered into the earth. I had been told that the worms would eat him. 'Slowly,' they said, but that the worms would eventually eat him up and, soon enough, there would be nothing left of his body. I couldn't understand this. Worms didn't have teeth. What superpower did they have to suck the flesh off our bones when we were vulnerable and alone inside the cold ground?

The crowd was quiet as we stood around the trench in the earth. I guess I believed them when they told me he was in that box being lowered into the earth; I had no reason not to. We trust a lot of people in our lives to tell us the truth. I guess he was in there, but I can't ever be sure. Not really. If he had been someone like Elvis then maybe we would have wanted so much for him to have somehow escaped that box that we'd make up stories about seeing him at the local milk bar. But I never saw my grandad again.

When I knew him, he was already an old man. He wore a flannel shirt, thick knitted jumpers and old suit pants. He picked carrots from his garden for us to eat as we headed home after our summer holidays with him and my nana. There were strict instructions that we were to eat the carrots, with dirt still stuck to them, once we had made the four-hour drive and were finally crossing the bridge near our home.

Eating a raw carrot was the last thing I wanted to do after four hours of driving. I would hold the carrot in my hand tightly enough so that if I drifted off to sleep, none of my siblings could prise it from my clutches. We were slammed together in that Holden HJ driving over dirt roads, and I was usually in the middle of two others in the back seat. But such was my dedication to the ritual that every time we reached that bridge and paid the twenty-cent toll, I would lift the carrot to my mouth and bite down.

Whenever I was a child I could only think of him as his thick skin and yellow teeth – I couldn't imagine him as bones and nothing, no matter how hard I tried. That the body I was in would one day find itself in a hole that had been dug for me was impossible to understand. I could think myself there as a basic concept, but not feel myself there. How was it possible to be nothing? The hole I would end up in wasn't going to be dug by a child who was trying to find her way to the other side of the world. Mine would be a hole dug by spades or perhaps a machine.

For all the life I had lived, all the ways I had lived upon the earth, I would be in the ground as bones and nothing for much longer. Just like the ash tree in Norse mythology, I would eventually find my way, as we all eventually did, to connect the world above and the world below.

Buddhists practise Maranasati, which basically translates as a meditation on death. It's a contemplation on the truth that everything that arises will eventually fall away so the human mind might begin to conceive the impermanence of all things and come to understand that change and death are the only things we can truly know. Contemplating our inevitable death is an attempt to quench the desires we have for this human form to exist perpetually so that we may begin to live more fully in the face of it all.

The Buddha is said to have had this reflection on ageing and death: 'If I – who am subject to ageing, not beyond ageing – were to be horrified, humiliated, and disgusted on seeing another person who is aged, that would not be fitting for me. As I noticed this, my young person's intoxication with youth entirely dropped away … If I – who am subject to death, not beyond death – were to be horrified, humiliated, and disgusted on seeing another person who is dead, that would not be fitting for me. As I noticed this, my living person's intoxication with life entirely dropped away.'[1]

* * *

When we were young it was impossible to comprehend how we might age and then die. Trying to understand that slowly, slowly, our cells break down or that we will dry up and lose our elasticity, that our entire system would weaken and die. How could that be when we felt so strong? So permanent. So unbreakable.

I was in the back seat of a car being driven by my boyfriend's best mate, Darren, or Daz, or Dazza, or Dazzé. He had somehow got his hands on his mum's maroon Holden, a model from the nineties, I think. He picked us up with a proud smile, sitting behind the wheel in his baggy jeans with a long mop of dark hair. We all knew that he battled with his demons, I guess, but none of us had any idea at that stage what we should do with that sort of information. He had told my boyfriend at the time that he knew he would die when he was young. So I guess we became bystanders, watching on, hoping nothing bad would happen to him – only capable of witnessing the innocence and darkness that would flash across his face in a constant light show.

I felt small around him. Not because he was one of those guys who dominated a room, but because he was in some ways so naive and otherworldly, and also because he was constantly on drugs. I didn't know how to act around him. He was polite and pretended to be interested in me, but I was surplus to his requirements. I spent most of my time watching his awkward, shy ways. But he loved my boyfriend, Phil, who loved him back just as much. And I loved him too, I guess, in the way you might come to love someone that you've watched intently from afar.

I spent my time spying on these two friends. It was the type of friendship made by two boys who loved each other simply. A love that is so fundamental and simple that it's never questioned, it just is. In any case, I was satisfied being ignored as I watched them laugh and insult each other, or try to out-rap the solos of songs in his tape deck.

There was something freeing about being with Darren, because around him I could pretend that I was like him, carefree and unafraid. I would roll my eyes at him in mock disapproval, but it was just a game and that was the part I was supposed to play. I trailed along behind in the wake of his complete disregard for the laws of physics, his refusal to acknowledge the lessons we had been taught about how to avoid death, and his belief that death would not come for him unless he agreed to its terms.

That afternoon, as we listened to something nineties on the tape deck in his mum's car, he took us into the backstreets of a leafy eastern suburb and, without warning, pushed hard on the accelerator. He didn't seem to care that we were in the car with him as he sped down a long, narrow suburban street. I wanted to scream but knew that might make the situation worse. I saw my boyfriend tense and grab at his arm. 'Darren,' I said, not sure what I wanted to say, not convinced that anything I could say would slow him down. And I wondered, as the houses blurred past us, what it would be like to die like this.

We were definitely hitting somewhere around 120 kilometres when, without much warning, we were flying. Just for the briefest moment. But even this many years later, I can freeze the movie on that bit. The bit when we are in the air. The thrill. The fear. The absurdity of it all. How unbreakable he must have thought we all were. For him, it must have been impossible to conceive of us in any other way. We were eternal. And we could fly.

When we landed back down with a thud, the steering wheel momentarily spun wildly out of his hands. But he slowed the car down and threw his hand up to high five one of us, but we were too scared to move.

Not long after, he killed himself. I can't remember the details. Funny that I remember when he made the car fly, but

I can't remember how he died. Phil wasn't my boyfriend when Darren died, so I didn't know quite how to mourn his death. I got dressed on the day of his funeral and sat on the edge of my bed, willing myself to be brave enough to go. I didn't feel like I had any right to be part of his life anymore, and now, no right to his death. So instead, I undressed and went to bed.

I have often wondered if he was hoping it might happen that day in the car. Did he want it to happen when we were having fun? Or did he really not see death the way I did, hard and immovable and real? For Darren, death wasn't something that happened to him, but instead something he knew he would have the final say on.

I wonder what he would look like now. He would be older than us, just a bit. What would he make of getting old? But he isn't old. And we can't imagine him that way because he froze that boy in time on the day he died. He didn't age like we all had, the ones he left behind.

Darren didn't see risk like I did. He didn't see the danger in our bodies, how they were fragile. How they would end and be broken somehow. He didn't think about that stuff, I don't think. On the other hand, I was someone who lay awake at night worried about how I would die. As a child I would write eulogies for my parents and have nightmares that their lives would end in a horror smash and they would never return home. I imagined it being up to me to speak at their funerals and tell the world who they were. I can't imagine how as an eight-year-old I would have spoken about death. I only understood it as the most frightening disappearance, an event cloaked in terror. I had seen it in movies, where there were tears and drama. I would rehearse how I would feel when the phone call came through. I would sometimes cry, practising my feelings like a method actor might. And I would make plans for what I would need to do to survive without them. Who would I like to live with and how would I look after my brothers and sister?

The fear started with my daydreams of death and then later when I slept, fear pulsing through my dreams. I guess I was trying to be ready for the bad things that could happen.

* * *

Father Patrick looked down at us from his pulpit. We were tiny, when I think back, and I was a believer. Year 3 was a big one for a Catholic – there's reconciliation, where you admit your sins, and then first communion, when you can finally eat bread and drink wine in the name of Jesus. Father Patrick's fat lips tripped over the words that spilled from him, still dripping in his saliva. His sermons were notorious for this; I was once spat on from about four metres away and wondered if it was a sign, perhaps, that I had been marked. His voice rumbled through his large frame. Maybe that day he was telling us about purgatory, the place you would go when God wasn't sure if you were good or bad. But it was very clear from what he had told us over the years that we would be punished for our sins. And we had undoubtedly all sinned.

I would pray with my eyes squeezed shut, begging that whatever I had coming, I would be let off total annihilation. 'Please don't take my family from me,' I pleaded. When I slid into the confessional booth I would rack my brains for any sin that I had perhaps committed. Even making one up was surely better than nothing if I wanted to clear my slate in the eyes of God.

The small wooden hatch separating the confessional booths would slide back and the breath of Father Patrick, heavy and acrid, would escape and fill my little room. His panting was laboured and sounded bored. He'd done this so many times before and my sins were paltry compared to others he must have heard. 'Bless me, Father, for I have sinned,' I would whisper, and probably sounded as if I very much meant it.

God spared me the death of my family, so the fear of death grew to a crescendo when I became sick in my mid-twenties. The imagined deaths of my family were suddenly replaced with my own. Nightmares were detailed and horrifying, and I would wake in the middle of the night gasping for air. In the dreams, I couldn't see or hear because darkness was all there was. I couldn't feel my body anymore, and the atmosphere seemed so heavy that when I tried to gulp in life, nothing could get through. In panic I was forced to burst out of my skin, to wake up my body from this sleep so I could breathe again.

While I was sick, death was a constant hum underneath my every day, a sense of dread that I would wake up with. Illness reduced my life in a way I imagine very old age takes the breath from you. Life becomes simple. Can I get out of bed? Can I walk to the sink? What TV show might I watch today? Will I be able to eat? And it reminds you that you are very fine glass, easily broken.

I was reading anything on death I could get my hands on, and one insight would lead me down a rabbit hole to find another. For a while I meditated every day, sitting for an hour at a time. Eventually, slowly, it changed me and my relationship with death.

* * *

We work to stave off the fear that death brings. To push back against its unrelenting promise. Over the last seventy years, the average life expectancy in Australia has increased by fifteen years to over eighty-three years. An extra fifteen years is a long time and a vastly different life with a vastly different set of expectations than those our grandparents might have had, who were dying on average in their late sixties and early seventies. And modelling suggests that by the time we hit 2100 we'll be living past ninety years of age.[2]

I have been walking through the local cemetery a lot lately. It is quiet and grand and ripe for contemplation. But it is full of the reminders of our ending. Of death. Of the importance we place in all these single lives. Lives that couldn't have imagined me walking past their graves a hundred years after they had died.

There are so many human lives buried in this cemetery who no one would know any longer. Their names would conjure no reaction from the people who have been left on this earth. Their memories do not inspire laughs or tears, but we are committed to honouring them with a patch of earth and a headstone. Living is the most important thing we do.

We try to make a mark on the earth while we are here. We try to make it so that it's hard to forget us. So that for years after we are gone, there will be people who will know that our lives had been worth living.

* * *

Ageing decay is often a sequential process where the body will break down in a certain order. The human body decomposes by eating itself. Our own 'decomposition begins several minutes after death, with a process called autolysis, or self-digestion'.[3] We have been built to finish it ourselves. We came alone, and we alone will ensure that we are entirely removed. We are hyper-alert to the signs of when it is beginning, to be ready to start the work to turn it back. To hold up our hands and demand that it should not happen yet. That it should slow or find another victim.

My son left an apple core on the bench. I decided that I wanted to watch it. The idea of watching something so still had never crossed my mind. I understood the idea of seeing the apple core on my bench, but to watch it was something else. To *watch* an apple core would be to understand it as somehow in motion, alive. Or perhaps, in the way I was thinking these days, it was in an active process of its death.

Moments ago it had been bright and delicious, its juice spilling over his chin. He was unconscious to the experience he was having, building Lego at the same time and barely aware that he was eating. He hadn't really noticed the beautiful life he was receiving from it. It was just an apple, after all. And he had left it on the bench because he wasn't really concerned with it now. As far as he cared, the apple was gone.

Most of us have little interest in this kind of decay that exists all around us. I wonder if it's been a way for us to ignore the death and decay that waits for us all. It is ugly, that's for sure. Perhaps this avoidance is an evolutionary reaction so that we won't consume death. We are revolted by the decay that lives around us. Of animals, of food, of our environment.

Perhaps this inability to see ageing and decaying as part of our own story is why we are so negligent of our environment. Perhaps this is why we cannot bear to look at the wholesale destruction that the human race is responsible for and why it makes us feel so bad. We are hell-bent on ignoring it for what it might mean to us more personally.

To be fair, my son wasn't the only one who had disregarded the apple. It wasn't something I had ever considered worthy of watching. Why would I spend time watching something so still? So ordinary.

The apple was only static relatively, and only because we insist on moving so quickly around such stillness do we fail to see the small changes taking place in our presence, the small deaths constantly on show. I had never taken the time to wonder about what it did when it was just there, on my bench.

So I decided to be a witness.

At first it glistened with the splendour of the devouring that had taken place. It was bright and alive, as if remembering that it had just been loved. But soon, within the space of an hour, it began to brown. The bruising was sporadic but swift, and the seeds that were once hidden now showed through the cracks. Birthing from the death of their host.

The science of it I had never bothered to wonder about.[4] I put the apple core on the teak buffet alongside other treasures and told everyone in the house not to throw it out. I brought it close to my face to see it from a new angle, dedicated to the task of being a worthy witness to its death. Trying not to be bored by the slowness of its change. Would I see it disintegrate? Where would it eventually go?

As the weeks passed, I counted the days as I always had, well rehearsed in my desire for the weekend. Hump day is Wednesday, the hardest day to endure because it's right in the middle between the last weekend and the one coming. Friday was usually the most enjoyable because you just had to get through it to get to the weekend. But then Monday was the first day of work week and I would dread it on Sunday, the last day of the weekend.

But the apple core had none of these markers. It experienced time as embedded into its DNA, an unavoidable reality of its biology. And as the weeks progressed, it slowly changed. Not as quickly as in those first few hours. But noticeably at least.

It became smaller and shrivelled and hard. It looked like it had endured years since the moment it had been devoured by my son and had shown the love of its life force. Now it was inedible. And discoloured. Dark and turning in on itself.

I kept watching.

In my own life, I was wishing and counting the days away but also had the audacity to wonder how the year had begun to feel as if was moving too fast. Too fast and also too slow, the sense of time we create from our deeply subjective perception of it.

And like this apple core, the human body has an incredible ability to 'interact with and alter the ecology of its wider environment. It is understood that our dead bodies are teeming with life',[5] and to imagine this changes the way I am beginning to think about my own death. My own decomposition. The body that is left behind will provide life beyond me.

In death we might know the true nature of our being, and that we return to the earth and continue to feed it brings me comfort. It helps me understand what the mystics always speak of: we are the earth, we are the sky, we are the wind, we are the water. So to return to it in a way that will then feed new life makes sense. There is no real ending.

* * *

I received a text the other day from Mat. We had met when I was about fifteen years old. He wore black jeans and a red button-down shirt with his long hair tied back into a low ponytail. We were in a group of mutual friends going to see a movie. Afterwards I tried to make small talk with him about the film; there was something about him I immediately liked.

Our friendship grew over the years through our shared love of both music and mucking around. The enormous luxury of friendship when you are young is the hours dedicated to each other and to play with no pressure of families to feed or real jobs to attend. Friendships at that age were one of our main occupations. It was a fundamental and pure time of ourselves when we were raw and real and we loved each other. As much as everything has changed, deep down I am the girl now that I was then.

Mat and I shared friends and food and parties and stages of our lives and talked about partners and annoying jobs. We also shared a mid-century home in Carlton North where we cooked soups and curries and vegetarian feasts. Next door lived an aggressive QC who would knock on our door screaming for Mat to stop playing his saxophone. And we would creep around hoping not to wake the heroin addicts who also shared the house or the very angry hippie whose suspicion and contempt of everything around him grew as the days rolled on.

When I saw Mat recently, I told him I remembered what he was wearing when we first met. He seemed surprised that I'd noticed him in the group that day – we had barely spoken. But there must be people you notice the first time you meet, because somehow you know they are going to be important in your story.

His text message told us that he was dying. They had given him three months, maybe nine at most. He comforted the group he had written to and told them that he understood the news would be hard to hear. But then he told us that he wasn't done. 'I'm going to fight this motherfucker as hard as I can,' he wrote. I read that line again. He was going to fight the cancer that had leached through his body, seeping into organs and bones. His hope that there might be a way to turn this entire ship around was painful to read. Hope is painful when it is like this. But he knew this wasn't possible; it was just the kindest way he knew to tell us the news that he knew would break our hearts. That he would fight hard for us.

But the hope that we might be more powerful than the inevitability of age and cancer and death is what we share with each other. Our hope is the expression of the love that we have for our life and the way that we honour its importance. The way we tell those around us that we want to stay on this earth with them. That we are bound to them and the lives that we live here. That this life mattered. That those curries and soups mattered. That drinking wine and playing music together mattered.

We are told we are brave when we fight death or show courage against its creep. When we are survivors of cancer or of other diseases that want to claim our lives, we are celebrated.

But what about that time when we can't win? There will be a day when it will be counted as a loss for each of us. I asked Mat how he felt about dying when I was sitting with him the other day. It seemed an absurd question. Almost stupid. 'How do you bloody think he'd feel?' I silently berated myself. He told me he was scared of the pain but had accepted that he was going to die and found a sort of peace with it. And then it occurred to me: there is an utter courage in letting go. In laying down and surrendering. In that moment of grace in the face of everything to have found a way to acceptance.

His breath moved in and out slowly. As he concentrated on each one, I watched him and began to focus on those breaths too. I had been rushing to get there, but now that I was with Mat, there was nowhere to be but here with him. It was beautiful. When I think back on it now, it feels like it was bathed in a gold light. Of course, we need to be careful not to mythologise these moments, but there was something elemental. Essential. Perfect.

We spoke about the old days. We laughed and we cried and I remembered something I had read once that described life as a beautiful vibration that oscillates between joy and heartbreak. That the dance is both.

As much as I had dealt with death of other people I have loved, and however much I have meditated on it and I believe I feel ready for my own, every time we're left here without someone that we love is an immeasurable pain. I still can't account for how much the world alters and adjusts and shifts to accommodate when someone we love is no longer here.

How can we account for this sort of loss? While I was sitting with Mat that day watching him breathe in and out, I decided I didn't want to. While he was still here with me, breathing in and out, I wanted to travel on each breath with him. I wanted to be in his living and not in his imminent death. The loss of his life was something I would deal with later.

* * *

I have seen death a few times. I watched on quietly as my own death was shown to me through my experience of illness – my fragility, the unexpected ways that my body could suddenly betray me. When I was sick, I had a premonition of my bones in the ground, my flesh having been eaten away, because I understood that I was really just a whisper from death's embrace. That we all were.

I have also seen death – touched it tentatively as I prayed with my eyes squeezed shut that it wouldn't notice I was in its company – when I have birthed my own children. They made it safely, somehow, from somewhere way out there into this world. But I had come to understand that a safe birth was not guaranteed. In fact, this might be the most dangerous part of our life as we arrive dangling precariously on the high wire, no safety net for us to dramatically fall into. Nothing to hold us as we travel here all by ourselves.

The miracle of children arriving on earth is impossible to give language to. We don't understand enough to ever speak of it with any real authority. Yes, we mostly understand it biologically, but that is only a portion of what is going on when a child is born.

I thought about my childhood tree when I gave birth to both my children. As they were about to break through, I knew we were nowhere. We were between the worlds, not belonging to either as my tree did. Instead, we were stranded between the earth above and the earth below. There was the thinnest of membranes that separated us from these worlds and I knew that if we weren't careful, we might pierce through its fragile form and be lost.

That's what it really feels like. Birth is a dance with heaven and earth. With above and below. When you have seen death up close, you understand birth through this paradigm. That birth and death are in fact the same. The crossing in and the crossing out are the same. At both these moments in our lives, we are the tree, above and below simultaneously, alone.

A body is the home of everything we are. The whirring love that travels through every atom and makes us feel as if we could fly, the searing burn we can feel cut into our skin when we lose something we believe is precious – all of it is trapped inside the body. Under the skin, inside the organs. It flows forever inside our blood. And the children we birth are bestowed all of it too. We pass the love and the trauma of these physical lives from one generation to the next.

Earth

CHAPTER 17

Boötes Void: Liminality

WHEN I LOOK UP at the sky, I'm fairly sure I don't understand it. I haven't the capacity of mind to wrap it around the idea that the sky is not the same as what I would draw when I was child. That I was at the bottom of the page on the earth and the sky was at the top, coloured in blue. The idea that there are nothings in our universe like the Boötes Void, seems impossible. I cannot fathom a place, or a no place, of nothingness.[1]

I find silence difficult. I have been trained to fill it with words and encouragement. Silence in my line of work is a problem, but at the same time, I crave it. I want to travel through the universe to the most silent place of nothingness so that I might make my journey across to the other side.

* * *

A liminal space is one of transition. A nothing space and an everything space. It is a space full of possibility while also being a place of purposeful waiting. Derived from the Latin word *limen*, meaning threshold, it is a precipice where we stand ready to jump if we are indeed brave enough.

Older women and younger women share this liminality as we enter and exit shared space during our various transitions, and for this moment of liminality we are transitioning at the same time, through the same portal. Liminal space in ritual is the middle stage of the transition, the point at which you are not your former self but you are yet to be your transformed self. And it is in this between space, located just beneath the topsoil, that our ageing is a relative affair. It only really makes sense as a comparison.

On dating apps, men's desirability peaks at fifty years of age and women's at eighteen. Women on average reach their highest career earnings at forty-four.[2] It feels that this age gap becomes a visceral space that lives between women. A divide. A clear line separating the before and the after. More than for men, women are treated as only two types: young and old.

The most glaring moment of comparison, the most compelling argument for age, is when you look into the eyes of the young women who have entered the space that we have been inhabiting. Being seen through their eyes is disarming, possibly crushing. The space between young women and me is the same distance that I once felt with women who were older and trying to enter my world.

I found that on top of the pain of my erasure by the wider world, the most painful moment was when I saw myself mirrored in the eyes of young women, who looked at me with boredom or disdain or both. That first moment when a teenage girl rolls her eyes at you, disgusted by your form, is like being knifed.

And there is fire in those eyes. This is a warning shot to frighten you away from any expectation that you might have an intimacy or solidarity with them. They warn you off their territory. Do not step foot on this land. You are in their way. You have made a mess of the world they are now inhabiting.

I have seen teenagers shift their eyes. It's difficult to imagine it happening when they are children and their eyes glisten when they watch you. When my son was nine years old he promised me he wouldn't do it. 'I won't become a bad teenager, Mum. I promise.' It feels impossible that there could ever be a time when they might betray you. 'Does she hate you?' ask women with teenagers of each other. 'Like no one in my life before,' is the answer, full of tentative humour, laced with a real fear. We are told it will pass, but will it?

The teenage girl travels into a deep annoyance of our place in their lives that is mixed with a quiet hope that we won't go too far from them. It feels like there was a time that we changed places, like the swap that happens in *Freaky Friday*. But we don't swap lives exactly, it's just the fine balance of dynamics that swing around like currents when the tide changes.

They take the lead, and we stand watching as they blaze ahead. It's a swift dethroning. It feels as if you have been cut down by the allies inside your own army at a time when you least expected it. At a time when you need them most. There is no more true unveiling than that which is done by young girls looking through the artifice of our older forms. They know us well enough, they have been cast in our image, so they know that to see through us is the fastest way to kill us and emancipate themselves from us.

Virtually overnight I became that same old woman who once watched me. And like the old women before, in front of young girls, I made it seem as if this process of becoming a woman was just a fun game. You close your eyes and squeeze your hands tightly and hope it won't be the same for them as it was for you. You tell them it's a beautiful thing, becoming a woman. And you make a joke of their experience of this change. 'Who are you trying to look pretty for?' you ask. 'Do you like someone?'

Because it hurts too much to tell the truth. Of the violence. Of the way our bodies felt heavy and hurt. Of how they held us back while we imagined we were being propelled forward. Of the ancient secrets of humiliation and being burnt and cut and drowned. Of how we've been unloved.

When the older woman and the younger woman intersect, this first instance is about the negotiation of the space that sits between us, that space of transformation. The space where we once rebelled and raised our voices and came together as young women, sure that we knew how to change the world.

I have been in awe of how younger women have taken the fight further. They have digested it and understood it more thoroughly than I feel we ever did when I was growing up. It has been fascinating to see my generation of women struggle to accept the ideological moves that younger generations are making. We have lived in their likeness but in a different time and space; they have new ideas and they're difficult to hear.

I always found it tough to see some older feminists misunderstand crucial changes in the world around them. You would hear violent ideas from someone who had been known as a grand warrior of the past, but now they were spouting notions that made no sense to us, saying there were only certain kinds of people who could be women. Or that younger women didn't know how to put up with the treatment that they had themselves endured: 'Suck it up, princess' was a refrain from the mouths of some women who once led the way.

It's an important process for a teenager to separate from the strong identities that have surrounded them and in part moulded them. The separation is essential in forming a self that can withstand an independent life. The moment when the child learns to fly is about finally seeing their body shadowed on the ground below them as a separate solid form. They are complete.

I see it in the teenagers who find their way into my home. Lounging on chairs and crammed tight into tiny bedrooms, they are weighed down by what they have been forced to believe they are. They are also carrying identities that have been struck with such force. And they are heavy with the tiresome job of trying to see themselves through all the murky images that are held up to them of who they should be.

But it's not simply about casting an independent form. It's about seeing the change they want to make in the world in themself. We are a reminder of how dangerous it can be to live as a woman, and a reminder that the world they have arrived in is dangerous. They have seen us being ridiculed. Being laughed at now for our oldness. But they share with us the experience of being in this world – they understand what we have come through because they see it now in them.

They can smell our desperation to remain important. Our existence annoys them. It is old and irrelevant. Surely they would see the fire that is still alive in me? Surely they would cut me some slack? This dethroning is harsh, possibly the harshest aspect of ageing.

Young women don't want to believe there is any way that we could in fact be a continuum, a part of them that has been propelled into another person in the future. It is unfathomable that we might somehow be connected to each other. But old women know we belong to each other – our lives just exist now in a different space and time. We know what lives inside those younger selves, the minds and hearts that beat with ferocity, because we have been them, we are them.

But we are taking up valuable space. Breathing valuable air. We are blocking a future that is demanding space to speak the way they see the world in their own voices, 'Shhhh,' they say when we speak too loudly, embarrassing them. They roll their eyes and look at you like you're the hysterical girl that you've always been told you are.

But did they understand that we fought for them? We are breathless in our indignation that they simply walked into the room, as if it had always been this way. What did they think we had been doing all these decades when we have been fighting for our lives? But they see it differently, as we did looking at the women whose footsteps we followed in.

And, it seemed, with one wave we had been erased from the place we felt we legitimately should take – sitting beside the women we had raised. The beheading is swift and definite. They want to run you out of town.

* * *

For a few weeks we were inundated by an idea that had begun circulating on social media: generation Z, the children of generation X, born in the late nineties, declared that it was embarrassing that older generations – millennials, Xers and boomers – still wore skinny jeans and side parts and used the crying emoji in text messages. Memes were constructed as the gen Z weapon of choice, and they took aim and fired relentlessly. Older women were ridiculed.

It seems petty to think of this as anything more than a playful jab from one generation to another, but it took on such a tone that it became clear that the youngster Zs wanted to own the older generations in a way that had never really happened before. They were unafraid to 'play the man', so to speak. So unrepentant was the attack that older women looked fearfully at each other. Women went out and bought straight-leg jeans so as to avoid the 'old' criticism that was being levelled at them. Millennials stopped combing their hair to the side.

The Zs had found the kryptonite of the generations that had gone before them: they used their age against them. They knew that fear of becoming irrelevant was the ultimate key to their undoing, and they realised they had all the power to proclaim what was now important. And old people were clearly not.

This intergenerational roasting wasn't new. The millennials had engaged in serious warfare with the boomers. At least in that battle, the millennials, armed with the hashtag #okboomer, were basing the attack around ideological issues like environmental crises and inequitable economic distribution of resources. But when it came to generation Z, the premise for this attack seemed to be based on the irrelevance of anyone older than them.

It had happened too when the boomers were young and they railed against the generations that went before them, demanding the world be a better place for those to come. They fought against wars and for the emancipation of women and people of colour and for sexual liberation.

What was strange about the gen Z attack was that they seemed unconcerned with fighting the generations before on ideological grounds and went straight for the jugular. This was about a grab for power – a taking over from the generations before them and asserting their place in the hierarchy. And they understood that to do so wasn't about arguing points of economic equity or how to save the earth from climate change. The Zs understood that this was about vanity and a desperate desire for the older generations not to be seen as old. As soon as they had us there we were begging them to call off the dogs.

In speaking to some gen Zs, they have argued that this warfare is more desperate than that of generations in decades gone by. Mali, born in the early 2000s, explains that this ruthless grab for power was done in the shadows of a world that looked like it was in its last throes. 'You have given us shit,' she says. 'You have had no regard for the world – the climate, the people who are vulnerable in every facet of this society, and we're here now having to clean up the mess you've made.' She laughed at my assertion that gen Z was more concerned with how we looked. 'You've got it wrong. We know that's what you care about. We're more than you think we are ... we're just not in the mood to play nicely, I guess.'

It became clear to me that assessments of generation Z had been made with the same basis of ignorance as those made of all the generations who had gone before. This wasn't a generation who had no idea but rather one that cared a lot and was just sick of a discussion that didn't lead anywhere. Those in power were still patently negligent when it came to the environment and continued to show blatant discrimination towards women, people of colour and other marginalised groups in society.

It occurred to me, finally, that my refusal to cede space and dismissal of the younger generation as being built on empty ideas is the same issue that women have faced for an eternity. If it wasn't men unwilling to give away their power and make space, it was older women, and usually older white women. I realised this time of liminality was more about my preparedness to show grace to the generations that were coming in after me. To show a humility to the young women in my life. To afford them an opportunity to be heard and make mistakes. To truly understand that they had something valuable to teach me rather than an arrogance of believing that my age meant I always knew better.

Becoming an elder and not just getting older, I realised, was going to be about this transition to listener. There was more for the world to gain if I became someone who learnt rather than someone who taught.

And so I decided that I needed to cede my place. The feminism looked different from the feminism I was used to; it had a militant edge that I know these women were working out how to navigate. But my role now was to listen, learn and support. It was time for me to move to the back of the room and know that moving there and holding that space was as golden as any of the spaces I had taken up before. If I had finally made my way to inside the gates, it was my job now to find a way to get other women in.

If there was anyone we wanted to do any of it for it was them, the beautiful girls we know ourselves to be, with beating hearts and ferocious minds who we know should take on this world. We want them to see themselves in our old bodies and feel proud, not frightened. When we are lost, so are they. The denial of our age is an erasure of our entire experience. It's a condoning of the abuse that we have endured since we were old enough to wear a flowery singlet top down to the shops to buy some chips.

I was starting to understand that getting older was the most important thing I could do. I needed to look upon the young women in my life with the eyes that had not looked upon me. Eyes that were able to see beyond the artifice and into that ferociously beating heart and mind.

ELEMENT:

Aether

New Beginnings

Aether

New Beginnings

I REALISE, AS I come to an end, that there is no neat ending to the question of age.

I am not new. I am the continuation of a certain kind of story. A story that has been on an eternal loop. I have been subjected to the same fate as women before me: to be lost on this earth. And then to be found again, but different – changed.

I am the girl who walked to the shops; she is me. This oldness that I am embarking upon is happening to that very same little girl. She is not gone. She is flowing through my blood. And each time I imagine her as someone else, something different, trapped in a photograph taken long ago and now stuck in a book, I lose the compass that I need to guide me through this. In the same way, every time I imagine that I am not the women who lived thousands of years before me, or who are yet to be born, I am lost. We are eternal; we are interchangeable.

What is the absolute elemental pure truth of this experience, this ageing process? How can we understand it so that we can understand ourselves properly, not necessarily in line with what the world wants from us? After all, surely by now we know we cannot trust the world. In the process of thinking about age I have started to face the pain of what it has meant to live as a woman. The understanding that I'm connected to the women that have existed well before me. The ones who were burnt and tortured and raped and hurt. And the ones who were loved and nurtured and that loved themselves. We are born and we die on an eternal loop. The world we are born in and live in has not changed, not really. It still seeks to kill us if we don't comply.

My meditation on age has been merely a series of questions. And I realise that while I began imagining I might find answers, in fact the job has been about finding the right questions to ask, questions that do not immediately demand an answer. I understand now more than ever that the first response to a good question should be to sit. And listen. And wait to hear what the answer might be, told to you through the earth, the wind, the fire and the water.

I had heard that I would disappear. I had heard about this kind of vanishing trick that women did. But as I start this disappearance, I wonder if I might leave the tiniest ripple. Will I be seen just a second before I am gone? Perhaps a little girl might catch me from the corner of her eye. 'Did you see that?' she might whisper. And it could be just enough for her to wonder if there was something out there, moving in the water, in the air, in the earth.

As we age, we become the wind, silently moving through town, barely raising the hairs or the eyes of any warm body that we pass. The natural world still loves us, though, and can still feel our weight as we walk upon it. We can see our footprints making a mark, heavy in the mud. 'I hope I have not entirely evaporated or transformed to vapour and cannot feel the world around me anymore' is a new daily mantra.

But where once we knew ourselves as strong, upright, stretching at full tilt into the sun, we soon come to understand that we are also ourselves even when we crouch to protect ourselves from the storms. None of us are immune from the human condition of death – of course we are not. And we must reconcile ourselves to the experience of ageing. But we finally come to understand ourselves through our broken and decaying forms because *we live here too*. We are unchanged inside, and that is the greatest trick of them all. The changed outer doesn't need to have any bearing on the interior life.

I call this the great expanse of the forever self.

Aristotle suggested a fifth element that later became known as aether. Evolved from the theories of his teacher Plato, he described aether as the essence of the universe, the stuff that filled the void and kept the universe in place.

Distinct from the oxygen humans were breathing on earth, the ancient Greeks proposed that aether was the air that the gods breathed in the heavens, personified by the Greek god Aether, who was one of the primordial gods of light and the sky. Aristotle theorised that aether transcended the earthly elements and gave the universe its ability to exist eternally.

Alchemists in the twelfth and thirteenth centuries believed that the other four elements – fire, air, water and earth – were transmutable and subject to change. But aether, the most pristine and divine element, was unchangeable. These medieval alchemists called it quintessence, and it was seen as the essence of elemental perfection.[1]

The forever self, then, is our perfect state – it is our elemental form. Our quintessence.

And so I wait in a limbo, in the liminal space, with my sisters, my ancestors, to gather strength for the next part of the journey.

Quiet, quiet, gentle, gentle.

But the fire still burns within me.

Dial up the wild. Unlatch the door. Flip the metaphoric table and rage until the last drop of all this has been birthed from you.

Then sit quietly, with your middle finger extended, and tell them to wait until you're ready.

And I'm not ready yet.

Endnotes

Prologue

1   Quoted in Caroline Baum, 'The ugly truth about ageism: It's a
    prejudice targeting our future selves', *The Guardian*, 15 September 2018:
    theguardian.com/lifeandstyle/2018/sep/14/the-ugly-truth-about-
    ageism-its-a-prejudice-targeting-our-future-selves.

Chapter 1

1   Lauren Lancaster, 'Street harrassment survey reveals girls as young as
    11 catcalled and followed', ABC News, 22 May 2018: abc.net.au/
    news/2018-05-22/street-harassment-survey-reveals-girls-as-young-as-
    11-catcalled/9783316.

2   Kari Walton and Cody Pedersen, 'Motivations behind catcalling:
    Exploring men's engagement in street harassment behavior', *Psychology
    & Sexuality*, 2021, DOI: 10.1080/19419899.2021.1909648.

3   Ibid.

4   Interview with Danny Blay, 8 September 2021. Danny Blay is a policy
    advisor and trainer in preventing family violence and violence against
    women and children. Danny was the chief executive officer of the No
    To Violence Male Family Violence Prevention Association.

5   Interview with Aakanksha Manjunath, 16 August 2021. Aakanksha is the
    Executive Director and co-founder of It's Not A Compliment.

6   Interview with Natasha Sharma, 26 August 2021. Natasha is a researcher and data analyst at It's Not a Compliment.

7   Callander D, Wiggins J, Rosenberg S, Cornelisse VJ, Duck-Chong E, Holt M, Pony M, Vlahakis E, MacGibbon J, Cook T. (2019). The 2018 Australian Trans and Gender Diverse Sexual Health Survey: Report of Findings [PDF], Sydney: The Kirby Institute, UNSW Sydney.

8   Australian National Research Organisation for Women's Safety Limited (ANROWS), 'Very few places where trans women of colour feel safe from abuse', 18 June 2020: anrows.org.au/media-releases/very-few-places-where-trans-women-of-colour-feel-safe-from-abuse/.

9   Interview with Natasha Sharma, 26 August 2021.

10   Leonard Sloane, 'Boom and bust on Wall Street', *New York Magazine*, vol. 1, no. 28, 14 October 1968, pp. 32–3.

11   Gillian Frank and Lauren Gutterman, 'How the "girl watching" fad of the 1960s taught men to harass women', *Jezebel*, 8 October 2020: jezebel.com/how-the-girl-watching-fad-of-the-1960s-taught-men-to-ha-1844916738.

12   Yeoman Lowbrow, 'A creepy 1959 guide to girl watching', *Flashback*, 21 March 2017: flashbak.com/a-creepy-1959-guide-to-girl-watching-376167/.

Chapter 2

1   Russell Brand, 'WAP with Cardi B and Megan Thee Stallion: Feminist masterpiece or p★rn?', YouTube, 14 August 2020: youtube.com/watch?v=EdP9H60N2l8.

2   Wendy Squires, 'Sorry, folks, but this is not the fresh new face of feminism', *Sydney Morning Herald*, 28 August 2020: smh.com.au/culture/music/sorry-folks-but-this-is-not-the-fresh-new-face-of-feminism-20200827-p55q0h.html.

3   Interview with Jessica, September 2021.

4   Steven Daly, 'Britney Spears: Inside the mind (and bedroom) of America's teen queen', *Rolling Stone*, 15 April 1999: rollingstone.com/music/music-news/britney-spears-inside-the-mind-and-bedroom-of-americas-teen-queen-188483.

5   Bianca Betancourt, 'Britney Spears speaks out about the *Framing Britney Spears* documentary for the first time', *Harper's Bazaar*, 31 March 2021: harpersbazaar.com/celebrity/latest/a35990365/britney-spears-reacts-to-framing-britney-spears-doc.

Chapter 3

1   Erique Zhang, 'The radical act of invisibility on Trans Day of Visibility', *The Washington Post*, 31 March 2022.

2   S. Liddel MacGregor Mathers, 'Of the experiment of invisibility, and
        how it should be performed', *The Key of Solomon the King* (Clavicula
        Salmonis), p. 51, 1888: sacred-texts.com/grim/kos/index.html.

Chapter 4

1   C.G. Jung, *Four Archetypes: Mother, Rebirth, Spirit, Trickster*, Princeton
        University Press, Princeton, NJ, 1970.
2   Joyce Tyldesley, 'Isis', *Encyclopedia Britannica*: britannica.com/topic/Isis-
        Egyptian-goddess.
3   Misa Han, 'Peter Costello's "baby bonus" generation grows up',
        Australian Financial Review, 1 Sept 2017: afr.com/politics/peter-costellos-
        baby-bonus-generation-grows-up-20170831-gy7wfgg.
4   Isabelle Roskam, Joyce Aguiar, Ege Akgun et al., 'Parental burnout
        around the globe: A 42-country study', *Affective Science*, no. 2, 2021,
        pp. 58–79: doi.org/10.1007/s42761-020-00028-4.
5   Ibid.
6   Interview with Steph, 3 October 2021.
7   Interview with Lois Peeler, 28 February 2022.
8   Australian Law Reform Commission Pathways to Justice – Inquiry into
        the Incarceration Rate of Aboriginal and Torres Strait Islander Peoples,
        2018, Australian Government.
9   Department of Health 'Clinical Practice Guidelines: Pregnancy Care:
        29.1: Family Violence', Canberra, (2020), Australian Government
        Department of Health.
10   Ibid.
11   Laila Tyack, 'Stolen at Birth: The painful legacy of Australia's forced
        adoption policy', *Vice*, February 2017: vice.com/en/article/evgxx7/
        stolen-at-birth-the-painful-legacy-of-australias-forced-adoption-
        policy.
12   Summeya Ilanbey 'Andrews government announces redress scheme for
        forced adoptions', *The Age*, 10 March 2022: theage.com.au/politics/
        victoria/abhorrent-then-condemned-today-andrews-government-
        announces-redress-scheme-for-forced-adoptions-20220310-p5a3ey.
        html#:~:text=He%20was%20one%20of%20250%2C000,of%20
        those%20adoptions%20were%20forced.

Chapter 5

1   Joseph Williams, 'Discover the truly grim history behind the fairy
        tale of Hansel and Gretel', *All That's Interesting*, 30 October 2021:
        allthatsinteresting.com/hansel-and-gretel-true-story.

2   Rebecca Beatrice Brooks, 'The witchcraft trial of Sarah Good', History of Massachusetts blog, October 2011: historyofmassachusetts.org/sarah-good-accused-witch/.

3   Ibid.

4   Bernard Rosenthal, *Salem Story: Reading the Witch Trials of 1692*, Cambridge University Press, Cambridge, 1993.

5   Sara Jobe, 'Sarah Good', Salem Witch Trials: Documentary archive and transcription project, 2001: salem.lib.virginia.edu/people/good.html.

6   Rebecca Beatrice Brooks, 'The witchcraft trial of Sarah Good', History of Massachusetts Blog, October 2011: historyofmassachusetts.org/sarah-good-accused-witch/.

7   James Massola, 'Julia Gillard on the moment that should have killed Tony Abbott's career', *Sydney Morning Herald*, 23 June 2015: smh.com.au/politics/federal/julia-gillard-on-the-moment-that-should-have-killed-tony-abbotts-career-20150622-ghug63.html.

8   Madeline Miller, 'From Circe to Clinton: Why powerful women are cast as witches', *The Guardian*, 7 April 2018: theguardian.com/books/2018/apr/07/cursed-from-circe-to-clinton-why-women-are-cast-as-witches.

9   David Kroll, 'The origin of witches riding broomsticks: Drugs from nature, plus Shakespeare', *Forbes*, 31 October 2017: forbes.com/sites/davidkroll/2017/10/31/the-origin-of-witches-riding-broomsticks-drugs-from-nature-plus-shakespeare/?sh=4f1feb2a61a9.

10 Marion Gibson, 'The witch: The facts behind the folktales', *The Conversation*, 15 March 2016: theconversation.com/the-witch-the-facts-behind-the-folktales-56233.

11 Pam Grossman, *Waking the Witch: Reflections on Women, Magic and Power*, Gallery Books, New York, 2019.

12 Julia Gillard, 'The "misogyny speech"', 9 October 2012: juliagillard.com.au/the-misogyny-speech/.

Air: Introduction
1   Tim Thwaites and Robert Whitehead, '35 years ago: A freak dust cloud envelopes Melbourne', *Sydney Morning Herald*, 7 February 2018.

2   Samantha Dick, 'On this day: A catastrophic dust storm engulfs Melbourne in 1983', *The New Daily*, 8 February 2021.

Chapter 6
1   Cassandra Szoeke, 'Healthy ageing program', The University of Melbourne: medicine.unimelb.edu.au/research-groups/medicine-and-radiology-research/royal-melbourne-hospital/healthy-ageing-program.

2   Jane Sims, 'Healthy ageing', *Australian Family Physician*, vol. 46, no. 1, January–February 2017.

3   Chloe Kent, 'From grinders to biohackers: Where medical technology meets body modification', *Medical Technology*: medical-technology. nridigital.com/medical_technology_jan20/from_grinders_to_ biohackers_where_medical_technology_meets_body_modification.

4   Sigal Samuel, 'How biohackers are trying to upgrade their brains, their bodies – and human nature', *Vox*, 15 November 2019: vox.com/future- perfect/2019/6/25/18682583/biohacking-transhumanism-human- augmentation-genetic-engineering-crispr.

5   Wim Hof, 'Why we breathe', Wim Hof Method: wimhofmethod.com/ breathing-exercises.

6   Bum Jin Park, Yuko Tsunetsugu, Tamami Kasetani, Takahide Kagawa and Yoshifumi Miyazaki, 'The physiological effects of *Shinrin-yoku* (taking in the forest atmosphere or forest bathing): Evidence from field experiments in 24 forests across Japan', *Environmental Health and Preventive Medicine*, vol. 15., no. 1, June 2009, pp. 18–26.

7   Interview with Lisa Leong, 9 March 2022.

Chapter 7

1   Carla Joinson, 'Loneliness too much to bear', Healing, hell and the history of American insane asylums, 28 October 2018: hhhasylum.com/ tag/prairie-madness/.

2   Lyall Watson, 'A brief eerie history of how the wind makes us crazy', *Lit Hub*, 13 August 2019: lithub.com/a-brief-eerie-history-of-how-the- wind-makes-us-crazy/.

3   Jacinta Parsons, 'Dealing with the shock of getting older', ABC Everyday, 23 April 2021: abc.net.au/everyday/dealing-with-the-shock-of-getting- older/100086632.

4   John Crace, 'Surviving the midlife crisis: A 10-point guide', *The Guardian*, 30 September 2010: theguardian.com/society/2010/ sep/29/10-point-guide-to-beating-that-midlife-crisis.

5   Interview with Anjali, Melbourne, November 2021.

6   Amy Capetta and Olivia Muenter, '17 signs you're having a midlife crisis', *Woman's Day*, 8 April 2021: womansday.com/health-fitness/ wellness/g2966/signs-of-midlife-crisis-in-a-woman/.

7   Elliott Jaques, 'Death and the mid-life crisis', *The International Journal of Psychoanalysis*, vol. 46, no. 4, 1965, pp. 502–14.

8   Ferdi Botha, 'Australia, are you OK? Here are the groups with the highest (and lowest) life satisfaction', *The Conversation*, 20 November

2020: theconversation.com/australia-are-you-ok-here-are-the-groups-with-the-highest-and-lowest-life-satisfaction-150363.

Chapter 8

1   Phil Edwards, 'Why people never smiled in old photographs', *Vox*,
    7 October 2016: vox.com/2015/4/8/8365997/smile-old-photographs.

2   Katy Kelleher, 'The ugly history of beautiful things: Mirrors', Longreads,
    July 2019: longreads.com/2019/07/11/the-ugly-history-of-beautiful-things-mirrors/.

3   Oscar Wilde, *The Picture of Dorian Gray*, Broadview Press, Peterborough,
    1998.

4   Benjamin Ramm, 'What the myth of Faust can teach us', BBC,
    26 September 2017: bbc.com/culture/article/20170907-what-the-myth-of-faust-can-teach-us.

5   Vanessa LoBue, 'Who's that baby in the mirror?', *Psychology Today*,
    10 February 2020: psychologytoday.com/au/blog/the-baby-scientist/202002/whos-baby-in-the-mirror.

6   Joshua A. Krisch, 'Five stages of self-awareness explain what babies see
    in the mirror', *Fatherly*, 27 October 2021: fatherly.com/health-science/children-five-stages-self-awareness-mirror-tests/.

7   Kim Eckhart, 'MEG used to measure infant brain responses to touch',
    Neuroscience News and Research, 17 January 2018: technologynetworks.com/neuroscience/news/meg-used-measure-infant-brain-responses-to-touch-296423.

8   Barbara L. Fredrickson and Tomi-Ann Roberts, 'Objectification
    theory: Towards understanding women's lived experiences and
    mental health risks', *Psychology of Women Quarterly*, vol. 21, issue 2,
    pp. 173–206: doi.org/10.1111%2Fj.1471-6402.1997.tb00108.x.

9   Tomi-Ann Roberts and Patricia L. Waters, 'Self-objectification and that
    "not so fresh feeling": Feminist therapeutic interventions for healthy
    female embodiment', *Women and Therapy*, vol. 27, no. 3, pp. 5–21,
    doi:10.1300/J015v27n03_02.

10 Jia Tolentino, 'Where millennials come from', *The New Yorker*,
    27 November 2017: newyorker.com/magazine/2017/12/04/where-millennials-come-from.

11 Gail Deutsch and Meghan Moore, 'Meet the mirror-free bride: Woman
    avoided mirrors for one year', ABC News, 15 August 2012: abcnews.
    go.com/Health/meet-mirror-free-bride-woman-avoided-mirrors-year/story?id=17003595.

12 Melissa Blake, 'After an internet troll told me I was "too ugly", I spent
    a year posting selfies', *Refinery29*, 30 September 2020: refinery29.com/

en-ca/2020/09/10063530/melissa-blake-writer-twitter-selfies-trollgate-
interview.

13 Melissa Blake, 'So about what I said …': melissablakeblog.com/about-
me.

14 Melissa Blake, 'After an internet troll told me I was "too ugly", I spent
a year posting selfies', *Refinery29*, 30 September 2020: refinery29.com/
en-ca/2020/09/10063530/melissa-blake-writer-twitter-selfies-trollgate-
interview.

15 Melissa Blake, Twitter, 3 February 2022: twitter.com/melissablake/
status/1489115890935283713?lang=en.

Chapter 9

1 Royal Meteorological Society, 'The Beaufort Scale': rmets.org/
metmatters/beaufort-scale.

2 Funmi Fetto, 'The beauty industry is still failing black women',
The Guardian, 29 September 2019: theguardian.com/global/2019/
sep/29/funmi-fetto-happy-in-my-skin-beauty-industry-diversity.

3 Lenny Ann Low, 'I want people to see me': Carly Findlay on rethinking
beauty, *Sydney Morning Herald*, 22 February 2020: smh.com.au/lifestyle/
beauty/i-want-people-to-see-me-carly-findlay-on-rethinking-beauty-
20200221-p5433f.html.

4 Damien Gayle, 'Facebook aware of Instagram's harmful effect on teenage
girls, leak reveals', *The Guardian*, 15 September 2021: theguardian.com/
technology/2021/sep/14/facebook-aware-instagram-harmful-effect-
teenage-girls-leak-reveals.

5 Leah Kozee, 'Unequal beauty: Exploring classism in the western beauty
standard' [thesis], Georgia State University, 2016.

6 Michelle Smith, 'The ugly history of cosmetic surgery', *The Conversation*,
29 April 2016: theconversation.com/friday-essay-the-ugly-history-of-
cosmetic-surgery-56500.

7 Department of Health, Health Workforce Data: Plastic Surgery, 2017,
Australian Government: hwd.health.gov.au/resources/publications/
factsheet-mdcl-plastic-surgery-2016.pdf.

8 Michelle Smith, 'The ugly history of cosmetic surgery', *The Conversation*,
29 April 2016: theconversation.com/friday-essay-the-ugly-history-of-
cosmetic-surgery-56500.

9 Health Science Degree, '10 Vintage Medicine Ads Selling Dubiously
Beneficial Products', Health Science Degree Guide, 25 April 2013:
health-science-degree.com/10-vintage-medicine-ads-selling-dubiously-
beneficial-products/.

10   Richard Ashby-Leeds, 'Cosmetic surgery ads divided by class', *Futurity*, 13 April 2012: futurity.org/cosmetic-surgery-ads-divided-by-class/.

11   Ashley Fetters, 'What's the point of long eyelashes?, *The Cut*, 30 April 2018: thecut.com/2018/04/the-psychology-behind-why-we-like-long-dark-eyelashes.html.

12   Mike Sacks, 'Justine Bateman doesn't want you to call her new book brave', *Vanity Fair*, 9 April 2021: vanityfair.com/style/2021/04/justine-bateman-doesnt-want-you-to-call-her-new-book-brave.

13   Sarah Berry, '"Whatever you need to do is fine" but ageing, sex and beauty co-exist', *Sydney Morning Herald*, 6 November 2019: smh.com.au/lifestyle/health-and-wellness/whatever-you-need-to-do-is-fine-but-ageing-sex-and-beauty-co-exist-20191105-p537jk.html.

14   Katie Couric, 'Is ageism getting old?', *Next Question* with Katie Couric, 31 October 2019: omny.fm/shows/next-question-with-katie-couric/is-ageism-getting-old.

15   Hunstad/Kortesis/Bharti Cosmetic Surgery, The normalisation of plastic surgery – don't be ashamed of your cosmetic surgeries': hkbsurgery.com/the-normalization-of-plastic-surgery.

16   Jaclyn S. Wong and Andrew M. Penner, 'Gender and the returns to attractiveness', *Research in Social Stratification and Mobility*, vol. 44, June 2016.

Chapter 10

1   Tessa Koumoundouros, 'Fish have "talked" for 155 million years, and now you can hear their "voices"', Science Alert, 5 February 2022: sciencealert.com/fish-have-been-talking-with-delightfully-strange-sounds-for-at-least-155-million-years.

2   Australian Human Rights Commission, Respect@Work: Sexual Harrassment National Inquiry Report (2020): humanrights.gov.au/our-work/sex-discrimination/publications/respectwork-sexual-harassment-national-inquiry-report-2020.

3   Webster, K., Diemer, K., Honey, N., Mannix, S., Mickle, J., Morgan, J., Parkes, A., Politoff, V., Powell, A., Stubbs, J., & Ward, A.: 'Australians' attitudes to violence against women and gender equality'. findings from the 2017 National Community Attitudes towards Violence against Women Survey (NCAS) (Research report, 03/2018). Sydney, NSW: ANROWS.

4   Stephanie Boltje and Annika Blau, 'Why do so few sexual assaults result in convictions?', ABC News, 14 November 2018: abc.net.au/news/2018-11-14/why-do-so-few-sexual-assault-result-in-convictions/10492256.

5   After the first trial ended in a mistrial, one man was found not guilty
        on four charges of rape and the jury could not reach a verdict on a fifth
        charge, which prosecutors later dropped. The second man was convicted
        of rape, but this was overturned on appeal. Elise Kinsella, 'In the witness
        box: How a court case put the spotlight on sexual assault trials', ABC
        News, 18 July 2021: abc.net.au/news/2021-07-18/how-a-court-case-
        put-the-spotlight-on-sexual-assault-trials/100281894.

6   Elise Kinsella, 'In the witness box: How a court case put the spotlight on
        sexual assault trials', ABC News, 18 July 2021: abc.net.au/news/2021-
        07-18/how-a-court-case-put- the-spotlight-on-sexual-assault-
        trials/100281894.

7   Callander D, Wiggins J, Rosenberg S, Cornelisse VJ, Duck-Chong E,
        Holt M, Pony M, Vlahakis E, MacGibbon J, Cook T. 2019. The 2018
        Australian Trans and Gender Diverse Sexual Health Survey: Report
        of Findings. Sydney, NSW: The Kirby Institute, UNSW Sydney. DOI:
        10.26190/5d7ed96ceaa70.

Chapter 11

1   Darcey Steinke, 'No one told me exactly what to expect from
        menopause. But the messages I did get were very wrong', *Time*,
        28 June 2019: time.com/5616247/menopause-expect-messages/.

Chapter 12

1   Franziska Alesso-Bendisch, 'Millennials want a healthy work-life balance.
        Here's what bosses can do', *Forbes*, 23 July 2020: forbes.com/sites/
        ellevate/2020/07/23/millennials-want-a-healthy-work-life-balance-
        heres-what-bosses-can-do/?sh=46ba84337614.

2   Australian Government, *Age Discrimination Act 2004*, Federal Register
        of Legislation.

3   Emma Dawson, 'Most poor people in the world are women. Australia
        is no exception', Per Capita, 7 May 2019: percapita.org.au/our_media/
        most-poor-people-in-the-world-are-women-australia-is-no-
        exception/.

4   Marianna O'Gorman and Emma Dawson, 'Superannuation: For
        women about to leave the workforce, the news isn't great', ABC News,
        31 August 2018: abc.net.au/news/2018-08-31/superannuation-it-is-
        time-to-close-the-gender-pay-gap/10174028.

5   Australian Government, 'Unpaid care work and the labour market',
        Workplace Gender Equality Agency, 2016: wgea.gov.au/publications/
        unpaid-care-work-and-the-labour-market.

6   Workplace Gender Equality Agency, 'Unpaid care work and the labour
     market' [insight paper]: wgea.gov.au/sites/default/files/documents/
     australian-unpaid-care-work-and-the-labour-market.pdf.

7   Sally Whyte, 'Forcing single parents on to Newstart has saved
     budget $5b, but increased poverty', *Canberra Times*, 6 March 2020:
     canberratimes.com.au/story/6650793/forcing-single-parents-on-to-
     newstart-has-saved-budget-5b-but-increased-poverty/.

8   Dinah Lewis Boucher, 'Female and homeless: Australia's growing
     housing crisis', *The Urban Developer*, 9 March 2021: theurbandeveloper.
     com/articles/female-homeless-australias-housing-crisis.

9   Ruth Quibell, 'A precarious place: Older women, housing insecurity
     and homelessness', *Women's Agenda*, 31 March 2019: womensagenda.
     com.au/life/a-precarious-place-older-women-housing-insecurity-
     homelessness/.

10   Maree Petersen and Cameron Parsell, 'Older women's pathways out of
     homelessness in Australia', The University of Queensland Institute of
     Social Science Research, Mercy Foundation Report, 2013.

11   National Older Women's Housing and Homelessness, 'Retiring into
     Poverty: A national plan for change: Increasing housing security for
     older women', Mercy Foundation, 2018: mercyfoundation.com.au/
     wp-content/uploads/2018/08/Retiring-into-Poverty-National-Plan-
     for-Change-Increasing-Housing-Security-for-Older-Women-23-
     August-2018.pdf.

12   Maree Petersen and Cameron Parsell, 'Older women's pathways out of
     homelessness in Australia', The University of Queensland Institute of
     Social Science Research, Mercy Foundation Report, 2013.

13   Andrew Hornery, 'No women members allowed: The Australian Club
     votes to remain open to only men', *Sydney Morning Herald*, 15 June 2021:
     smh.com.au/lifestyle/gender/no-women-allowed-the-australia-club-
     votes-to-remain-open-to-only-male-members-20210615-p5813r.html.

14   Ibid.

15   Tikka Jan Wilson, 'Feminism and Institutionalised Racism: Inclusion
     and exclusion at an Australian Feminist Refuge', *Feminist Review 1*,
     doi:10.2307/1395769.

16   Sarah Hill, 'A lack of intersectional data hides the real gender pay gap',
     Women's Agenda, 28 August 2020: womensagenda.com.au/latest/a-lack-
     of-intersectional-data-hides-the-real-gender-pay-gap/.

17   Ruby Hamad, *White Tears/Brown Scars*, Melbourne University Press, 2019.

18   Aileen Moreton-Robinson, *Talkin' Up to the White Woman: Indigenous
     Women and Feminism'* (20th anniversary edition), University of
     Queensland Press, 2 July 2020.

Chapter 13

1   Daniel H. Pink, *The Power of Regret: How Looking Backward Moves Us Forward*, A&U Canongate, February 2022.

2   Nancy E. Newall, Judith G. Chipperfield, Lia M. Daniels, Steven Hladkyj and Raymond P. Perry, 'Regret in later life: Exploring relationships between regret frequency, secondary interpretive control beliefs, and health in older individuals', *International Journal of Aging and Human Development*, vol. 68, no. 4, pp. 261–88.

3   Stephen Dark, 'Britain was the first to appoint an official minister for loneliness in 2018 – what's going on?', *The Fifth Estate*, 8 March 2021: thefifthestate.com.au/urbanism/publiccommunity/britain-was-the-first-to-appoint-an-official-minister-for-loneliness-in-2018-whats-going-on/.

4   Tony Pagone QC and Lynelle Briggs AO, Final Report: 'Care, dignity and respect', Royal Commission into Aged Care Quality and Safety, 1 March 2021: agedcare.royalcommission.gov.au/publications/final-report.

5   Jacinta Parsons, 'Amid the chaos of COVID-19, heart-warming text messages remind us of the value of friendship', ABC Radio Melbourne, September 2020: abc.net.au/news/2020-09-25/friendships-shine-despite-distance-of-covid-19-pandemic/12692652?nw=0&r=Image.

Earth: Introduction

1   Patti Wigington, 'Ash tree magic and folklore', Learn Religions, 23 December 2018: learnreligions.com/ash-tree-magic-and-folklore-2562175.

Chapter 14

1   Interview with Lois Peeler, 28 February 2022.

2   Nina V. Guno, 'Woman engaged to husband again after forgetting him due to brain injury', Inquirer.net, 23 August 2019: newsinfo.inquirer.net/1156796/woman-engaged-to-husband-again-after-forgetting-him-due-to-brain-injury.

3   Elizabeth Loftus and Katherine Ketcham, *Witness for the Defense: The Accused, the Eyewitness, and the Expert who Puts Memory on Trial*, St Martin's Press, New York, 1991.

4   Rachel Aviv, 'How Elizabeth Loftus changed the meaning of memory', *The New Yorker*, 5 April 2021: newyorker.com/magazine/2021/04/05/how-elizabeth-loftus-changed-the-meaning-of-memory.

Chapter 15

1   C.F. Carver, 'The mask we wear: Chronological age versus subjective "age inside"', *International Journal of Aging Research*, 2(1), 29: doi. org/10.28933/ijoar-2019-02-2606.

Chapter 16

1   Eugene Cash, 'The Paradox of Maranasati Practice', Spirit Rock: An Insight Meditation Center, 2021: spiritrock.org/the-teachings/article-archive/the-paradox-of-maranasati-practice.

2   'Australia life expectancy 1950–2022', Macrotrends: macrotrends.net/ countries/AUS/australia/life-expectancy.

3   Mo Costandi, 'Life after death: the science of human decomposition', *The Guardian*, 5 May 2015: theguardian.com/science/neurophilosophy/2015/ may/05/life-after-death.

4   Lynne McLandsborough, 'Why do apple slices turn brown after being cut?', *Scientific American*, 30 July 2007: scientificamerican.com/article/ experts-why-cut-apples-turn-brown/.

5   Mo Costandi, 'Life After Death: the science of human decomposition', *The Guardian*, 5 May 2015: theguardian.com/science/neurophilosophy/2015/ may/05/life-after-death.

Chapter 17

1   George Dvorsky, 'Behold the Boötes void, the spookiest place in the cosmos', *Gizmodo*, 6 July 2012: gizmodo.com/behold-the-bootes-void-the-spookiest-place-in-the-cosm-5923493.

2   Maya Salam, 'For online daters, women peak at 18 while men peak at 50, study finds. Oy.', *New York Times*, 15 August 2018: nytimes. com/2018/08/15/style/dating-apps-online-men-women-age.html.

Epilogue

1   Meg Neal, 'The eternal quest for aether, the cosmic stuff that never was', *Popular Mechanics*, 10 February 2021: popularmechanics.com/science/ energy/a23895030/aether.

References

'Ash Wednesday bushfires: 16 February 1983', ABC News: abc.net.
au/news/emergency/2013-02-14/ash-wednesday-bushfires-
1983-from-the-archives/4519214?nw=0&r=Map.

David Kroll, 'The origin of witches riding broomsticks: drugs
from nature, plus Shakespeare', *Forbes*, 31 October 2017:
forbes.com/sites/davidkroll/2017/10/31/the-origin-of-
witches-riding-broomsticks-drugs-from-nature-plus-
shakespeare/?sh=4f1feb2a61a9.

Acknowledgements

Firstly, to the women I can feel in my blood and who have blazed this trail – to my mother and my grandmothers, thank you.

I also want to dedicate this book to our beautiful Mat Baulch – you taught me, more than anyone else could, about how to live by sharing with us the utter grace of your death.

And to Claire, your wife, I feel lucky to love you and to be your earth ball™.

To my partner, AJ, who has believed in and supported me so that I could actually write this book, thank you for your love and your faith and your patience. To my little legs, Perry, you are wise beyond your years and give good advice – thank you for those 'five' transcendent hugs. And to Mika, you are one of my greatest loves and scored the dedication so I will use this space to ask you for my black cords back.

Thank you to the inimitable Catherine Milne for creating

this book with me. Your belief and energy and humility is the reason I found these words. I wrote this because you asked me to, because you knew there was a story here. I hope you are proud of what we made.

To everyone at HarperCollins and ABC books – especially Simone Ford for a cracking edit, Barbara McClenahan for your support and Sandy Cull for a stunning cover.

The BIGGEST of thanks to my book doula Monica Dux for your unwavering advocacy, kindness, support and brilliant mind. Thank you for the early readings of this work and for our many, many walks around the cemetery in contemplation of these ideas and our death, and for the hours we spent wondering why you decided to learn German. And for sharing an interest in finding where the mafia is buried both literally and metaphorically. You are an incredible human, and I am indebted.

To Rita Moclair, who was one of the great women. In your memory, thank you for everything you gave me.

To the whip-smart Yves Rees, who was beyond generous with their time, insight and care with a sensitivity read of this book – I am so grateful.

To the fiercely brilliant women who read this book early for me: Peggy Frew, Mimi Kwa, Julia Zemiro, Veronica Gorrie, Nyadol Nyuon and Monica Dux. And to the #punk Clare Bowditch. I learn so much from all of you – thank you.

Every day of the work week I get to kick out with some of the strangest and most wonderful people – my Afternoon family on the ABC. You are the creative force in my life and a constant reminder of what is truly beautiful. Thank you for everything you have taught me.

To my work peeps, especially Jo and John for putting up

with me every. single. day. and John for arguing for 12 months with sustained passion about the merits (or otherwise) of reality television celebrities. I am right.

To Dina, Shelley, Mary-Jane, Warwick, Kon and Sally for supporting me to extend my wings while keeping the wheels spinning at ABC Radio Melbourne – thank you so bloody much.

To my manager and compadre Lena Barridge, who is simply wonderful. Above all, thank you for your friendship. You got me less drunk more often this time around – of which I am grateful. And to Henri Stride for all the support from the far reaches of Sydney.

To Matthew Parsons for the photos and to all the friends that I found my way back to during the writing of this book: Phil, Soraya, Romy and Anthony. And to Ineke, who has been standing beside me since that first bowl of hot chips and gravy 30 years ago – I love you. To my leggin'-clad Kate Blanchfield and to my new romance Martha – I love you both so much. Sorry for crying on your couch for two hours after you'd just given birth but thank you for your true love – I am so lucky. And Fi Pepps (and Charlie), I miss our daily hangs but thank you for your long-distance love.

To the Morries, always, Libby and Kirsty, who have sat with me on a Tuesday since the dawn of time. And to the big-up support of Daniel James, who encouraged this book with frequent word checks and insights – thank you also, for connecting me to some incredible women. And to Donna for becoming a spiritual hippy – finally – and for your endless support of me through some wild times.

Violet, what fortune it was that I stumbled across you in a laneway in Melbourne more than 10 years ago. You have been a light and a huge reason this book exists at all. Thank you so much for your guidance and friendship over all these years.

To Steph Hughes, even though your business card says 'workplace bully of Jacinta Parsons', I remain in awe of you. You are ridiculous. And joyous. And brave.

To my brain mums, Lisa Waller and Lucy Morieson from RMIT, who have encouraged this book and my creative work. And to the bloody ace crew of people who are sharing the PRS (explain to me what it's all about again …) 'journey', you are all very brilliant.

For the skillz of Nat Bartsch for creating the album *Hope*, which I listened to over and over while I wrote this book. Your music is woven through these pages (I hope that's okay!!).

And to all the people who contributed to this book with their ideas, research, stories, hearts and lives, I hope this is the beginning of a conversation that will honour you. Big thanks especially to Jessica, Carrie, Danny, Fiona, Lois, Steph, Lena, Anjali, Phil, Mat, Claire, Natasha and Aakanksha.